Business of Otolaryngology

Editors

STEPHEN P. CRAGLE
EILEEN H. DAUER

OTOLARYNGOLOGIC CLINICS OF NORTH AMERICA

www.oto.theclinics.com

Consulting Editor
SUJANA S. CHANDRASEKHAR

February 2022 • Volume 55 • Number 1

ELSEVIER

1600 John F. Kennedy Boulevard • Suite 1800 • Philadelphia, Pennsylvania, 19103-2899

http://www.oto.theclinics.com

OTOLARYNGOLOGIC CLINICS OF NORTH AMERICA Volume 55, Number 1
February 2022 ISSN 0030-6665, ISBN-13: 978-0-323-85007-0

Editor: Stacy Eastman
Developmental Editor: Diana Ang Grace

Otolaryngologic Clinics of North America (ISSN 0030-6665) is published bimonthly by Elsevier, Inc., 360 Park Avenue South, New York, NY 10010-1710. Months of issue are February, April, June, August, October, and December. Business and Editorial Offices: 1600 John F. Kennedy Blvd., Suite 1800, Philadelphia, PA 19103-2899. Customer Service Office: 6277 Sea Harbor Drive, Orlando, FL 32887-4800. Periodicals postage paid at New York, NY and additional mailing offices. Subscription prices are $450.00 per year (US individuals), $1336.00 per year (US institutions), $100.00 per year (US & Canadian student/resident), $576.00 per year (Canadian individuals), $1396.00 per year (Canadian institutions), $628.00 per year (international individuals), $1396.00 per year (international institutions), $270.00 per year (international student/resident). Foreign air speed delivery is included in all *Clinics'* subscription prices. All prices are subject to change without notice. **POSTMASTER:** Send address changes to *Otolaryngologic Clinics of North America*, Elsevier Health Sciences Division, Subscription Customer Service, 3251 Riverport Lane, Maryland Heights, MO 63043. **Telephone: 1-800-654-2452 (U.S. and Canada); 314-447-8871 (outside U.S. and Canada). Fax: 314-447-8029. E-mail: journalscustomerservice-usa@elsevier.com (for print support); journalsonlinesupport-usa@elsevier.com (for online support).**

Reprints. For copies of 100 or more of articles in this publication, please contact the Commercial Reprints Department, Elsevier Inc., 360 Park Avenue South, New York, NY 10010-1710. Tel.: 212-633-3874; Fax: 212-633-3820; E-mail: reprints@elsevier.com.

Otolaryngologic Clinics of North America is also published in Spanish by McGraw-Hill Interamericana Editores S.A., P.O. Box 5-237, 06500 Mexico D.F., Mexico.

Otolaryngologic Clinics of North America is covered in *MEDLINE/PubMed (Index Medicus), Current Contents/Clinical Medicine, Excerpta Medica, BIOSIS, Science Citation Index,* and *ISI/BIOMED.*

Contributors

CONSULTING EDITOR

SUJANA S. CHANDRASEKHAR, MD, FACS, FAAOHNS
Consulting Editor, Otolaryngologic Clinics of North America, Past President, American
Academy of OtolaryngologyeHead and Neck Surgery, Secretary-Treasurer American
Otological Society, Partner, ENT & Allergy Associates LLP, New York, New York; Clinical
Professor, Department of OtolaryngologyeHead and Neck Surgery, Zucker School of
Medicine at HofstraeNorthwell, Hempstead, New York; Clinical Associate Professor,
Department of OtolaryngologyeHead and Neck Surgery, Icahn School of Medicine at
Mount Sinai, New York, New York

EDITORS

STEPHEN P. CRAGLE, MD, FACS
Partner, St. Cloud Ear, Nose & Throat Clinic, P.A., St Cloud, Minnesota

EILEEN H. DAUER, MD, FACS
President, Partner, St. Cloud Ear, Nose & Throat Clinic, P.A., St Cloud, Minnesota

AUTHORS

WILLIAM R. BLYTHE, MD, FACS
Partner, East Alabama Ear, Nose and Throat, PC, Opelika, Alabama

RICHARD C. BOOTHMAN, JD
Boothman Consulting Group, LLC, Ann Arbor, Michigan, USA; Principal, Boothman
Consulting, Adjunct Assistant Professor, Dept. of Surgery, University of Michigan Medical
School, Visiting Scholar, Vanderbilt University School of Medicine, Center for Patient
Safety and Professional Advocacy Nashville, Tennessee

CAROL R. BRADFORD, MD, MS, FACS
Dean, College of Medicine, Vice President for Health Sciences, Wexner Medical Center,
The Leslie H. and Abigail S. Wexner Dean's Chair in Medicine, The Ohio State University
Wexner Medical Center, Columbus, Ohio

MICHAEL J. BRENNER, MD, FACS
Associate Professor, Department of Otolaryngology–Head and Neck Surgery, University
of Michigan Medical School, Ann Arbor, Michigan; GTC Quality Improvement
Collaborative, Durham, North Carolina

DAVID J. BROWN, MD
Associate Dean and Associate Vice President for Health Equity and Inclusion, Associate
Professor, Department of Otolaryngology–Head and Neck Surgery, Michigan Medicine,
Ann Arbor, Michigan

CRISTINA CABRERA-MUFFLY, MD
Associate Professor, Department of Otolaryngology–Head and Neck Surgery, University of Colorado School of Medicine, Aurora, Colorado

CHRISTOPHER Y. CHANG, MD
Fauquier Ear, Nose, and Throat Consultants, Warrenton, Virginia

STEPHEN P. CRAGLE, MD, FACS
Partner, St. Cloud Ear, Nose & Throat Clinic, P.A., St Cloud, Minnesota

JESSICA CRONIN, MD, MBA
Medical Director of Quality and Safety, Associate Professor of Surgery and Pediatrics, George Washington University School of Health Sciences, Children's National Hospital, Washington, DC

EILEEN DAUER, MD, FACS
President, Partner, St. Cloud Ear, Nose & Throat Clinic, P.A., St Cloud, Minnesota

D. SCOTT FORTUNE, MD
Allergy & ENT Associates of Middle Tennessee, PC, Hermitage, Tennessee

CARRIE L. FRANCIS, MD
Associate Professor, Department of Otolaryngology–Head and Neck Surgery, Associate Dean, Workforce Innovation and Empowerment, Faculty Affairs and Development, Kansas University Medical Center, Kansas City, Kansas

CHRISTINA M. GILLESPIE, MD
Partner, Ocean Otolaryngology, Toms River, New Jersey

KENNETH GRUNDFAST, MD
Professor, Department of Otolaryngology, Boston University, Boston, Massachusetts

SAMANTHA J. HAUFF, MD
Physician Owner, Sunset ENT, San Diego, California

HOSAI TODD HESHAM, MD
Adjunct Faculty, Department of Surgery, Division of Otolaryngology, George Washington University, Washington, DC; Maryland ENT Associates, Privia, Private Practice, Silver Spring, Maryland

KATHERINE HICKS, MD
Assistant Professor, Department of Otolaryngology–Head and Neck Surgery, UTMB Health, Galveston, Texas

GERALD B. HICKSON, MD
Joseph C. Ross Chair of Medical Education and Administration, Professor of Pediatrics, and Founding Director, Center for Patient and Professional Advocacy, Vanderbilt University Medical Center, Center for Quality, Safety and Risk Prevention, Vanderbilt University Medical Center, Nashville, Tennessee

ALEXANDER JIN
TPIU Foundation

LESLIE KIM, MD, MPH
Associate Professor and Division Director, Facial Plastic and Reconstructive Surgery, Department of Otolaryngology–Head and Neck Surgery, The Ohio State University Wexner Medical Center, Columbus, Ohio

SUSAN KOPREK
Front Desk Lead, St. Cloud Ear, Nose & Throat Clinic, P.A., St Cloud, Minnesota

K.J. LEE, MD, FACS
Donald and Barbara Zucker School of Medicine at Hofstra/Northwell; Quinnipiac University; Frank H. Netter MD School of Medicine; Yale School of Medicine; HaloMedia Group

LAWTON C. LEUNG, AB, JD, LLM
Attorney, Withers Bergman LLP, Private Client and Tax Team, New Haven, Connecticut

ANGELA LIESER
Director of Finance, St. Cloud Ear, Nose & Throat Clinic, P.A., St Cloud, Minnesota

JAMES LIN, MD
Associate Professor, Department of Otolaryngology–Head and Neck Surgery, Kansas University Medical Center, Kansas City, Kansas

ROBIN W. LINDSAY, MD
Department of Otolaryngology – Head and Neck Surgery, Harvard Medical School, Massachusetts Eye and Ear, Boston, Massachusetts

JAMIE R. LITVACK, MD, MS, FARS
Lead, Surgical Subspecialties, Department of Medical Education and Clinical Sciences, Elson S. Floyd College of Medicine, Washington State University, Everett, Spokane, Tri-Cities, Vancouver

SONYA MALEKZADEH, MD, FACS
Vice Chair, Education, Residency Program Director, Professor, Otolaryngology–Head and Neck Surgery, MedStar Georgetown University Hospital, Washington, DC

LANCE A. MANNING, MD, FACS
Chairman, Board of Governors, American Academy of Otolaryngology–Head and Neck Surgery, Adjunct Clinical Assistant Professor, Department of Otolaryngology, University of Arkansas for Medical Sciences

BRIAN McKINNON, MD, MBA, MPH
Associate Professor and Chair ad interim, Department of Otolaryngology–Head and Neck Surgery, UTMB Health, Galveston, Texas

MARK E.P. PRINCE, MD, FRCS(C), FACS
Charles J Krause M.D. Collegiate Professor and Chair, Department of Otolaryngology–Head and Neck Surgery, Rogel Cancer Center, University of Michigan Medical School, Ann Arbor, Michigan

RICHELLE REINHART, MD
Fellow, Neonatology, George Washington University School of Health Sciences, Children's National Hospital, Washington, DC

AMANDA RESSEMANN, CENTC
Business Office Lead and Certified Coder, St. Cloud Ear, Nose & Throat Clinic, P.A., St Cloud, Minnesota

CYNDA HYLTON RUSHTON, PhD, MSN, RN, FAAN
Anne and George L. Bunting Professor of Clinical Ethics, Johns Hopkins University School of Nursing, Department of Pediatrics, Berman Institute of Bioethics, Johns Hopkins University School of Medicine, Baltimore, Maryland

KATHLEEN SARBER, MD
Assistant Professor, Department of Surgery, F. Edward Hebert School of Medicine, Uniformed Services University of the Health Sciences, Bethesda, Maryland; Staff, Department of Otolaryngology–Head and Neck Surgery, Brooke Army Medical Center, Fort Sam Houston, Texas

RAHUL K. SHAH, MD, MBA
Vice-President, Chief Quality and Safety Officer, Professor of Surgery and Pediatrics, George Washington University School of Health Sciences, Children's National Hospital, Washington, DC

SUPARNA SHAH, MD
Fellow, Department of Otolaryngology–Head and Neck Surgery, Oregon Health & Science University, Portland, Oregon

ANDREW G. SHUMAN, MD, FACS
Associate Professor, Department of Otolaryngology–Head and Neck Surgery, Co-Chief Clinical Ethics Service, Michigan Medicine, Ann Arbor, Michigan

GARIN L. STROBL, JD
Constellation Mutual, Minneapolis, Minnesota

DALE AMANDA TYLOR, MD, MPH
Riviera ENT, Cottage Hospital Santa Barbara, Santa Barbara, California

RICHARD W. WAGUESPACK, MD
Member, CPT Assistant Editorial Board, CPT Advisor for the Triological Society, (Retired) Department of Otolaryngology–Head and Neck Surgery, The University of Alabama at Birmingham, Birmingham, Alabama

JULIE L. WEI, MD, FAAP
Division Chief, Pediatric Otolaryngology/Audiology, Director, GME Wellbeing Initiative, Nemours Children's Hospital, Chair, Otolaryngology Education, Professor, Otolaryngology–Head Neck Surgery, University of Central Florida College of Medicine, Orlando, Florida

Contents

joy in work. Part 3, Health Professional Wellness and Resilience, introduces the final pillar for advancing the clinical mission.

Making the Business Case for Quality and Safety

Rahul K. Shah, Richelle Reinhart, and Jessica Cronin

There is broad understanding and appreciation that quality and safety are indispensable parts of the business enterprise of delivering care. However, because health care organizations have resource constraints and competing priorities, leaders and managers must create, demonstrate, and articulate a business case for continuing to prioritize investments in quality and safety. To accomplish this, one must leverage financial principles with compelling story-telling. Success creates a virtuous cycle whereby ongoing investments in robust structures increase returns (value defined as improvements in quality and safety outcomes), and cost savings are reinvested to continue to improve delivery of high-quality care.

New Payment Models: The Medicare Access and CHIP Reauthorization Act of 2015, Merit-based Incentive Payment System, Advanced Alternative Payment Models, Bundling, Value-Based Care, Quadruple Aim, and Big Data: What Do They Mean for Otolaryngology?

Stephen P. Cragle

New payment models have been introduced by the Centers for Medicare and Medicaid Services to move medicine away from volume-based care toward value-based care. Most models focus on changes for primary care, but specialists like otolaryngologists are wise to familiarize themselves with this changing payment landscape to take advantage of the opportunities and avoid the pitfalls associated with each model.

Marketing Your Practice: Setting Yourself Apart in a Competitive Market, Online Reputation Building, and Managing Patient Experience/Satisfaction

Leslie Kim, Dale Amanda Tylor, and Christopher Y. Chang

The days of making a first impression when you meet your patients in person are numbered. Rather, in today's digital age, your prospective patients have likely already formed opinions about you and your practice before they meet you. And these opinions are largely influenced by the information they discover about you online. While you cannot completely control your personal brand or reputation as a physician, you can certainly try by controlling your online narrative: communicate your expertise and your value by effectively using social media, by regularly updating your practice website, and by proactively managing patient satisfaction reflected on physician rating websites. Set yourself apart in a competitive market today by building a strong digital presence.

Coding for Optimal Payment (Correct Coding 2022 for Otolaryngology)

James Lin and Richard W. Waguespack

The coding process can be confusing to medical professionals; understanding how to do so correctly will optimize reimbursement and keep the provider safe from potential economic and medicolegal problems.

This article reviews the coding and valuation processes and provides specific examples to aid the in how to correctly report procedures.

A perfect storm of events to include the COVID-19 global pandemic and technologic advances has led to the emergence of telemedicine in otolaryngology as a means to deliver remote clinical services to patients in their home and other clinical settings. There are benefits, such as increased safety and increased access to care, but also challenges, such as need for advanced technology and familiarity with computers. Telemedicine could play a greater role in otolaryngology in the future with advances in smartphone and endoscopic technology allowing for more detailed examination of patients.

This article relates the first-hand experience of a surgeon who faced 2 medical malpractice actions separated by 30 years and how each of those experiences affected him. The first episode occurred early in his career and caused anxiety, fear, and anger. The importance of getting support during a medical malpractice event, and the opportunities to do so, are discussed. The timeline of a typical medical malpractice lawsuit and phases of the litigation process are detailed. The authors provide guidance on how to make this process less stressful. The article summarizes medical malpractice lawsuits involving otolaryngologists.

To care for your family and to do "good" for your alma mater, religious organization, and the other charities you love, you need to do "well," which is to build a successful practice. To achieve a successful practice, following the principles of the dozen A's is helpful: Ability, Availability, Amicability, Approachable, Attuned, Aware, Attentive to patients, Attentive to others, Attentive to details, Apology (ability to apologize and accept apology gracefully), Assimilate, Affordable. Another way to put it is "skills to treat, heart to care at a sensible price."

The financial considerations of becoming a physician are often not fully understood or appreciated until after residency and fellowship training. Once training is complete, physicians face a combination of increased financial rewards mixed with significant, and seemingly overwhelming, financial responsibilities, often with limited financial knowledge or understanding. Appropriately managing debt obligations, living expenses, saving for retirement, children's education, and establishing financial safety nets through savings, investments, and insurance are critical. This article is a starting point to provide the new physician with an introduction into some of those financial considerations, to both encourage further learning and promote successful financial decisions.

As practicing clinicians, most of us have not had formal education on many of the business fundamentals that allow us to run a thriving practice. This article serves as a primer for understanding revenue cycle management, practical steps for engaging in insurance contract negotiation, and considerations for benchmarking the financial, operational, and human resources of your clinic.

Diversity impacts performance of our teams, fosters innovation, and improves outcomes of our patients in otolaryngology head and neck surgery. In addition to the moral imperative, increasing the otolaryngology diversity workforce will decrease health care disparities while equity and justice can increase the culture humility to take care of an increasingly diverse patient population. To move toward justice, otolaryngology departments need to end biases in faculty hiring, development, research evaluations, and publication practices. The more intentional our efforts, the more benefit to our patients, providers, staff, learners, and society.

OTOLARYNGOLOGIC CLINICS OF NORTH AMERICA

FORTHCOMING ISSUES

April 2022
Pituitary Surgery
Jean Anderson Eloy, Christina H. Fang and Vijay Agarwal, *Editors*

June 2022
Comprehensive Management of Headache for the Otolaryngologist
Joni K. Doherty and Michael Setzen, *Editors*

August 2022
Gender Affirmation Surgery in Otolaryngology
Regina Rodman and C. Michael Haben, *Editors*

RECENT ISSUES

December 2021
Childhood Hearing Loss
Nancy M. Young and Anne Marie Tharpe, *Editors*

October 2021
The Dizzy Patient
Maja Svrakic and Meredith E. Adams, *Editors*

August 2021
Biologics in Otolaryngology
Sarah K. Wise, Ashkan Monfared and Nicole C. Schmitt, *Editors*

SERIES OF RELATED INTEREST

Facial Plastic Surgery Clinics
Available at: https://www.facialplastic.theclinics.com/

Foreword

"Business" Is not a Four-Letter Word

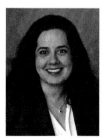

Sujana S. Chandrasekhar, MD, FACS, FAAOHNS
Consulting Editor

Remember back to when you decided you wanted to be a physician? You made the conscious decision to study instead of going out, to spend your weekends and evenings buried in books and memorization, maybe even foregoing that really interesting humanities course because you had to "ace" organic chemistry. You did this because you wanted to be a doctor to help people and make a difference in this world, and that's what you told your medical school interviewers. Me, too. Not one of us said, "I want to be a doctor and make sure I run my business profitably so that I can pay my staff and myself fairly and stay in business to continue to help more patients and provide for my family and retire comfortably." Likewise, our curricula in medical school were rich in basic and clinical sciences, and more recently in ethics and communication, but, all along training, information continues to be sparse regarding business basics, employment and insurance negotiations, the intricacies of human resource management, billing, coding and getting paid, what to do in case you are sued, and how to plan for your and your family's financial future. In fact, our students and trainees are often led to believe that it is somehow unseemly to view what we do as a business. That is wrong.

Most of the business lessons I have learned were acquired through trial and error, through realizing what I don't know, through educating myself, and through understanding that the word "business" as it applies to comprehensive, compassionate health care, is the third leg of the three-legged stool upon which our practices are built. A successful and rewarding Otolaryngology practice requires all three legs: having a deep knowledge of the existing *science* and steadfastly pursuing continuing medical education; paying close attention and giving importance to the *art* of understanding the patient and their family, respecting their cultural and medical customs and mores, and developing one's skills in communication and shared decision making; and, yes, dedicating oneself to understanding and optimizing one's *business*, be it as part of

Otolaryngol Clin N Am 55 (2022) xiii–xv
https://doi.org/10.1016/j.otc.2021.10.001
0030-6665/21/© 2021 Published by Elsevier Inc.

an academic enterprise, a large single- or multispecialty group, a governmental entity, or a small or solo practice. Having three strong legs not only allows the stool to support one's own practice but also permits us the time, space, and energy to deliberately shape the future of Otolaryngology so that it rightly reflects the patients and communities we serve.

Otolaryngologic Clinics of North America prides itself on identifying subjects within our field that are worthy of a dedicated issue for a comprehensive "deep dive" to benefit otolaryngologists and related colleagues in the United States, in Canada, and around the world. When Dr Stephen Cragle approached me with the idea of putting together a Business of Otolaryngology issue, I jumped at it. He and Dr Eileen Dauer have successfully drawn upon their wealth of knowledge and experience. They have assembled an outstanding treasure trove of articles by authors who themselves bring diverse and comprehensive reflections on each of their topics. The seventeen articles in this issue address topics that affect every aspect of our practices. They weave choice of practice type in with professionalism, pay equity, diversity, leadership, wellness, quality, and patient safety. There are terrific articles that explain the alphabet soup of new payment models and coding for optimal payment, incorporating telehealth, surviving litigation, and marketing your practice in an ethical manner while utilizing traditional and social media effectively. I hope you, the reader, take the time to read through each of them, as the lessons you will learn are truly priceless.

I congratulate Drs Cragle and Dauer on their passion for helping otolaryngologists understand the business of our profession. This issue of *Otolaryngologic Clinics of North America* gives the reader vital information while encouraging a mindset that moves from orphaning the business side of the practice, in effect, treating it as an unmentionable four-letter word, to bringing it in as that vital third leg of a stable and successful career in Otolaryngology.

www.ears.nyc

Sujana S. Chandrasekhar, MD, FACS, FAAOHNS
Consulting Editor
Otolaryngologic Clinics of North America

Past President
American Academy of Otolaryngology–
Head and Neck Surgery

Secretary-Treasurer
American Otological Society

Partner, ENT & Allergy Associates LLP
18 East 48th Street, 2nd Floor
New York, NY 10017, USA

Clinical Professor, Department of Otolaryngology–
Head and Neck Surgery
Zucker School of Medicine at Hofstra–Northwell
Hempstead, NY, USA

Clinical Associate Professor
Department of Otolaryngology–
Head and Neck Surgery
Icahn School of Medicine at Mount Sinai
New York, NY, USA

E-mail address:
ssc@nyotology.com

Preface

Minding Our Own Business!

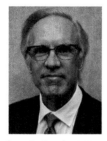   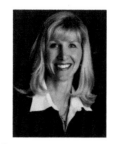

Stephen P. Cragle, MD, FACS   Eileen H. Dauer, MD, FACS
Editors

Modern health care practice is an art, a science, and a business. Regardless of practice type, academic, employed, or private, physicians find themselves faced with economic, financial, and management decisions the effects of which transcend the physician-patient relationship to broadly impact our economy and society. The art of medicine and the science of medicine are well represented in training programs, national meeting agendas, and continuing education courses, while the business of medicine is often left to on-the-job training, administrative briefings, and curbside discussions prior to department or board meetings. Apart from time- and resource-consuming formal Executive MBA Programs, there is a paucity of educational content with an emphasis on the business of medicine for the practicing physician. Yet there is tremendous value in understanding business basics, including general accounting principles, revenue cycle management, insurance contract negotiation, coding, new payment models, telehealth, and marketing.

In addition to understanding business basics, as we advance through our careers, we need to prepare for several important decisions: what type of practice should we pursue? What if we are unhappy with that choice, how do we change gears? How do we build and sustain a successful practice, and manage debt, investments, and estate planning? How do we become effective leaders? How do we support our patients when a complication arises? How do we promote a culture of patient safety within our practices and in the house of medicine more generally? How do we face the unpleasant circumstance of a malpractice claim? How do we effectively advocate for diversity and income equality within our specialty and beyond?

We are honored and excited to present this collection of articles from experts in the Business of Otolaryngology, and we are grateful for the diverse group of authors with whom we have had the privilege to work. We sincerely hope you find these articles

Otolaryngol Clin N Am 55 (2022) xvii–xviii
https://doi.org/10.1016/j.otc.2021.09.001
0030-6665/22/© 2021 Published by Elsevier Inc.

oto.theclinics.com

interesting and full of useful, practical tips that bring success and fulfillment to you in your career, wherever it may lead you!

Stephen P. Cragle, MD, FACS
St. Cloud Ear, Nose & Throat Clinic, PA
1528 Northway Drive
Saint Cloud, MN 56303, USA

Eileen H. Dauer, MD, FACS
St. Cloud Ear, Nose & Throat Clinic, PA
1528 Northway Drive
Saint Cloud, MN 56303, USA

E-mail addresses:
scragle@stcloudent.com (S.P. Cragle)
edauer@stcloudent.com (E.H. Dauer)

Twitter: @docsadvice (S.P. Cragle)

The Physician as Leader
Navigating the Breadth of Opportunity and Finding Your Best Fit

William R. Blythe, MD[a], Sonya Malekzadeh, MD[b,*], Julie L. Wei, MD[c]

KEYWORDS

- Physician • Leader • Leadership development • Education

KEY POINTS

- Many physicians take on leadership responsibilities over the course of their careers but may feel ill-prepared to lead.
- Leadership development is an important aspect of closing the leadership gap.
- Best fit opportunities for leadership should correspond to physician strengths and needs and position them for growth.

INTRODUCTION

As today's complex health care landscape continues to evolve, the leadership opportunities have grown exponentially. Strong and effective leaders are needed to cope with these challenges and who better to lead the effort than those with experience on the front lines? Physicians offer a unique perspective and can provide useful insight and information that stems from experiences as key members of the health care team.

The decision to take on a leadership role is an important one. Physicians must be prepared to put their own interests secondary to the interest of the rest of the entity. Great leaders live for something bigger than themselves, bigger than their dreams of personal fame, position, authority, or money. True leadership lies in coping with change and transforming a compelling vision into reality. Exemplary leaders have the ability to inspire and energize individuals, guide them to success, and ensure that everyone is performing at their best.

[a] East Alabama Ear, Nose and Throat, PC, 1965 1st Avenue, Opelika, AL 36830, USA; [b] Department of Otolaryngology-Head and Neck Surgery, MedStar Georgetown University Hospital, 3800 Reservoir Road, NW, Washington, DC 20007, USA; [c] Division of Pediatric Otolaryngology/Audiology, Nemours Children's Hospital, 6535 Nemours Parkway, Orlando, FL 32827, USA
* Corresponding author.
E-mail address: malekzas@georgetown.edu

Otolaryngol Clin N Am 55 (2022) 1–9
https://doi.org/10.1016/j.otc.2021.07.006
0030-6665/22/© 2021 Elsevier Inc. All rights reserved.

There is no formula or direct path to a leadership position and becoming an effective leader is an evolutionary process. Although some may aspire to these positions, many are thrust into roles of leadership. The key to success is early involvement and adequate preparation to develop those skills and qualities that will make us true leaders.

This article first reviews factors related to leadership development followed by a description of the different opportunities and pathways toward leadership, as described from 2 personal perspectives. The first focuses on issues relevant to leadership in private practice, whereas the second considers matters surrounding academic medicine.

LEADERSHIP DEVELOPMENT

At some level, all physicians are considered leaders. As surgeons, we "lead" everyday; the decision to go to the OR is an example of leadership. We have the ability to identify potential problems, anticipate the impacts of those challenges, and prioritize solutions. We know how to manage stress, get out of trouble, and are comfortable with the concept of accountability. We have a healthy fear of failure but know how to manage and learn from it.

Many physicians assume that these qualities coupled with the clinical experiences that have made us successful in solo practice or small team environments translate into leadership ability. Unfortunately, physicians receive little, if any, exposure to leadership training. We are taught to be independent problem-solvers and to develop authoritative decision-making abilities. To be effective leaders, we need to shift from being individual contributors focused on technical competence and clinical expertise to a large-picture, vision-oriented, and systems mindset (**Table 1**).

The key to overcoming these challenges is to learn. Just as physicians have to learn clinical expertise to practice medicine, they have to acquire a new set of competencies to master the practice of leadership. Leadership training equips physicians with 2 core sets of skills. The first centers on self-awareness and interpersonal abilities that include displaying emotional intelligence, building and coordinating teams, and interprofessional communication. A second, separate set of necessary skills deals with business intelligence such as finance, strategy formulation, change management, and systems thinking. This deeper understanding produces leaders who can handle the operational and administrative challenges in a variety of settings.

Physicians interested in furthering their leadership knowledge and capabilities can choose from a vast amount of information that is now available (**Table 2**). Over the past several decades, an ever-increasing number of offerings and experiences are available in the marketplace that provide specific content on health care and the physician's perspective as a component of their curriculum. Different training options will appeal to different audiences. These include certificate or degree programs, ranging from short online courses to in-person longitudinal curricula that allow more time for participants to practice the skills they are learning in their current environment. Today an ever-increasing number of physician leaders are graduates of business schools. Although an MBA does not guarantee a leadership position, the additional education provides the tools to speak the language of business, understand the complexities of health care delivery, and view the health care world from a practical vantage point.

The importance of a strong network of champions in leadership development cannot be underestimated. Mentors and sponsors can help navigate the path forward and serve as sounding boards. They can be critical in helping aspiring leaders gain the

Table 1	
Medicine versus Leadership	
The Nature of Medicine	**The Nature of Leadership**
Prescribe and expect compliance	Lead, influence, and collaborate
Immediate and short-term focus and results	Short-term, medium-term, and long-term focus and results
Procedures/episodes	Complex processes over time
Relatively well-defined problems	Ill-defined, messy problems
Individual or small focus	Larger groups crossing many boundaries, integrated approach
Being the expert and carrying the responsibility	Being one of many experts and sharing the responsibility
Receiving lots of thanks	Encountering lots of resistance
Respect and trust of colleagues	Suspicion of being a "suit"

From October 2012 issue of Trustee magazine, Vol. 65, No. 10 © 2012 by Health Forum Inc https://trustees.aha.org/sites/default/files/trustees/center-voices-10-12.pdf

perspective and connections they need to take on larger roles and advance their careers. Coaches can assist in areas where you might need improvement such as building confidence communication or presentation skills. Executive coaches can help with promoting and establishing yourself as a thought leader in a particular field.

PHYSICIAN LEADERSHIP IN PRIVATE PRACTICE (WILLIAM BLYTHE)

The development of physician leaders in private practice is a challenging endeavor. This is due in part to competing and conflicting interests in time, professional goals, and finances, but is also a function of differing attitudes and priorities of private practitioners. However, physicians in private practice serve in critical leadership roles that are essential to organized medicine.

The first steps toward leadership often begin within the physician's own practice, where they often build the foundations of expertise necessary for the endeavor. Medical school does not prepare physicians for business management, human resources, or legal expertise, so much of this must be learned through experience and effort. A busy medical practice offers an opportunity to learn the business of medicine from the roots up, and its success is critically dependent on the physician owner's participation and leadership. Whether in sole or large group practice, a strong physician leader must begin by ensuring that their own house is in order and successful. Seasoned and experienced physician partners are invaluable resources for education and experience.

Wider leadership opportunities often begin with the local hospitals and surgical centers. Credentials Committee is a sound foundational introduction to service and leadership, as it educates physicians in the foundations of medical staff service and privileges. Leaders should attend departmental meetings and offer service as needed and should volunteer for work and committees as those opportunities present. Leadership opportunities often present in sections and departments within institutions and are often the best places to begin the journey. Peer Review, Physician Health, Pharmaceuticals and Therapeutics, EHR and Technology committees always need interested members, and those are often good opportunities to serve and learn. After a physician has some experience and reputation with the medical staff, election to

Table 2 Leadership development tools and resources		
3.1 Courses		
Program	**Institution**	**Time Frame**
Surgeons as Leaders: From Operating Room to Board Room	American College of Surgeons (ACS)	Summer
Early Career Women Faculty Leadership Development Seminar	Association of American Medical Colleges (AAMC)	Summer
Mid-Career Women Faculty Professional Development Seminar	Association of American Medical Colleges (AAMC)	Winter
Minority Faculty Career Development Seminar	Association of American Medical Colleges (AAMC)	Fall
Leadership Program for Health Policy and Management	Executive Education Program, The Heller School for Social Policy and Management, Brandeis University	Summer
Leadership Agility Program	Society of University Surgeons (SUS) in collaboration with Kellogg School of Management	Fall
Constructive Collaboration: Driving Performance in Teams, Organizations and Partnerships	Executive Education, Kellogg School of Management, Northwestern University	Fall/Winter
3.2 Extended Opportunities		
Program	**Institution**	**Duration and Details**
Faculty Leadership Institute	The Ohio State University College of Medicine	Monthly courses, year-long
Brandeis Health Leadership Program (BHLP) in Health Policy and Management	Brandeis The Heller School for Social Policy and Management	1 wk session
Harvard Macy Institute		Various
Hedwig van American Executive Leadership in Academic Medicine® (ELAM®)	Drexel University College of Medicine	3 wk sessions
Leadership Academy	American College of Physicians	18 mo
Physician Leadership Program	Wharton School, University of Pennsylvania	3 courses over 9 mo
Women's Leadership Institute	UCLA Anderson School of Management Executive Education	Live, online over 3 mo

Medical Executive Committee and Medical Staff Officer positions are often a natural progression.

Civic and County medical societies offer additional opportunities to extend leadership outside of the local institution. Leadership often begins by simply attending the meetings, reading correspondence, and volunteering for opportunities to serve. County medical societies often report to the state medical society and BOME, and leadership opportunities abound from those connections. County and state medical societies often look for physicians with relationships or connections to legislators, as those connections often prove invaluable to the House of Medicine. As one gains experience, reputation, and connections, leadership opportunities at the state level often open.

Local and state specialty societies offer abundant opportunities for networking and developing leadership. Many physicians choose to focus their time and efforts within their own specialty or subspecialty, as those often have the most significant interest and direct effect on their practice. Commonly, physicians feel that the smaller the specialty society and the narrower the focus, the more pertinent a society is to them personally. This is true in many respects, especially if the physician has a very limited scope of practice. They often feel that the larger organizations do not represent or understand their circumstances well, so they tend to focus on their smaller area of interest.

This last statement is applicable to national societies and organizations as well. Physicians often become members of large professional organizations such as the AMA and ACS early in their careers, but later find them too large and generalized to be applicable to their practice. In many circumstances, physicians gravitate to specialty and subspecialty national organizations. This has the advantage of being more directly applicable to a limited practice, but has the disadvantage of small size, membership, and representation. The larger organizations have the professional and financial clout to have substantial lobbying power and institutional influence, and therefore maintenance of their membership is essential. Many physicians find leadership opportunities in the smaller national organizations first, and later migrate to positions of leadership and influence in the larger national organizations over time.

Physician leadership is foundational to the "traditional" model of health care, which is organized around an independent, self-governed medical staff within the medical practice, hospital, and other facilities. The key to this model is the term "self-governed," which is predicated on bylaws, rules, and regulations created by and for the medical staff. Typically, the general medical staff creates and approves bylaws, and the medical staff leadership creates and approves policies, procedures, and rules/regulations. They also set standards for credentialing and privileges of the medical staff, as physicians are in the best position to understand and regulate these very important aspects of medical practice.

Unfortunately, medical school does not specifically prepare physicians for organizational leadership, and those are skills that must be learned and refined. Any physician desiring to embark on leadership roles should strongly consider formal education and training in physician leadership skills. This training can be obtained through experience and mentorship, but is often best accomplished with formal leadership training. This is readily available for institution-based physicians, but must be specifically sought out by those in private practice. There are numerous private companies and academic institutions that offer leadership conferences and workshops, and those can be invaluable sources of education and practical leadership training. Leadership training can prepare physicians to be better prepared to avoid the many landmines that can be stepped on in the field of peer leadership. This is particularly important in credentialing and Peer Review.

It is also important for physicians—particularly those in private practice—to examine and consider their motivation and goals for endeavoring in leadership. Typically, a private practitioner's compensation and professional advancement is unaffected by leadership service, and if anything, it may take away from their professional practice. It is tempting to assume that leadership service allows the physician to earn the esteem, appreciation, and admiration of their family, friends, and colleagues, and that is certainly true in many circumstances. However, the job of the physician leader is to govern their colleagues and to make tough but firm decisions, and that is unappreciated and resented in many circumstances. It is an understatement to suggest that physicians, in general, do not value and appreciate critique and criticism. This is particularly in the face of adverse outcomes and disruptive behavior. It is the physician leader's responsibility to ensure that peer review and disciplinary meetings are conducted thoroughly and fairly. The best care and safety of the patient is always paramount, with fairness to the colleague and open disclosure being a close second. Leadership can be a thankless, unappreciated, and resented job, but someone has to take the responsibility of doing it. This is particularly true for those of us who value and desire to maintain self-governed, organized medical staff.

Leadership service places a significant time demand and stress on a good leader. Meetings and communication are almost always conducted after the busy clinical and surgical hours. Spending time and energy dedicated to leadership activities is a choice to spend those precious commodities away from friends and family. This can take a significant toll on personal relationships, family, and friends. There are only so many hours in a day, and a choice to spend those in one area is an active choice not to dedicate them elsewhere. These considerations must be weighed when measuring work-life balance.

However, it must be emphasized that physician leadership is an act of service—to one's peers, patients, and institutions. The reward for these efforts is in the service itself, similar to the reward of being a physician many times. As mentioned earlier, someone must fulfill these leadership obligations, and if not, our autonomy and influence over the delivery of health care will be taken away from us. For far too long physicians have allowed hospitals, insurance companies, and government to take control of health care and make the decisions that physicians are best able to make. This trend will only worsen if we do not continue to nurture and develop strong, thoughtful, pragmatic leaders who are best able to lead and advocate on behalf of patients and physicians.

PHYSICIAN LEADERSHIP IN ACADEMIC MEDICINE (JULIE WEI)

As I reflect on my career as a physician and physician leader since 2003, it is humbling how overwhelmed I was just to start my first "job" as an attending as a faculty of an academic otolaryngology department. I spent the next decade at the same institution, building clinical practice at both the tertiary children's hospital as well as a satellite office. In addition to growing surgical expertise in routine and complex cases, I devoted immeasurable effort to all things "academic": teaching during one-on-one interactions, didactics to trainees and all allied professionals, clinical research projects, submission of abstracts to various society meetings, writing manuscripts, among other activities. As the years went by, while juggling family and work, such activities also provided a rich network of relationships with colleagues within and outside my institution and across various subspecialties of Otolaryngology.

"Leadership" was not a concrete concept that I associated myself with. Upon reflection, I was engaged in too many activities in the name of "career-building." While I enjoy the fruits of my own labor, it came at the cost of my physical and emotional well-being, infertility, sacrificed time and energy away from loved ones, and resulted in a high degree of burnout without recognizing how I got there. Leadership from early in my career seemed defined by others who had "titles," division chiefs, department chairs, various "names" and "roles" that other physicians had in addition to their training in whatever subspecialty.

During the first decade of my career, I was frustrated by the lack of opportunities for career development as defined by "titles." It was after I had the opportunity to serve as the President of Women in Medicine and Science at our Medical Campus, leading not only physicians but basic scientists and countless female clinicians across the School of Medicine, School of Nursing, and School of Allied Health, that I realized the "power" and boundaryless influence one can make as a part of a greater group. Inspiring others and uniting talented individuals who share similar visions and goals to create positive change provided the greatest professional fulfillment above and beyond my daily role as a pediatric otolaryngologist. After 3 years, it was clear that I craved a change in my professional life, which would not only provide but mandate "leadership" in every aspect of the role. In the past 8 years, I am humbled to have helped recruit and build a talented team. We have established a huge footprint through our pediatric health system across Central Florida with immense access for children and families, created medical student clerkships and education, mentored and conducted clinical research, facilitated matching in otolaryngology, created GME wellbeing programs and initiatives for the medical staff, and countless other efforts that reflected my core values. During recent 3 years, I had the opportunity to serve as the Surgeon-in-Chief for our hospital, which provided immense opportunities for "leadership" in the creation, implementation, and alignment among surgeons, anesthesiologists, CRNAs, and perioperative and OR staff.

Leadership for me turns out to be the expression of one's principles through consistent behaviors, learning complexities of interwoven factors that impact other team member's daily experience, creating synergy and engagement to ensure the highest quality and safety for patient care in our daily performance. I have also learned that leadership is defined by how others experience you. Leaders make constant decisions that support the professional and personal fulfillment of those within their sphere of influence and beyond. One may be assessed as a "good" or "great" leader if those served "feel" absolutely trusted and supported without judgment, even when mistakes occur. As leadership for me is defined by behaviors, the possibilities in any practice setting and across subspecialties, within and outside a division/department/institution, become endless (**Table 3**).

For most, the perception and belief in oneself as a leader may require and/or be reinforced by a "title" or formal role as "leadership" is typically associated with the "authority" to function over others in any hierarchy. Understanding that leadership is primarily relational, achieved by social capital through trusted and deeper relationship with others, is what allows the ability to inspire and achieve shared goals while leveraging unique and various perspectives and strengths across any collaborative group for any purpose.

The topic of leadership skills is vastly described by numerous books and articles, but key skills include active listening, empathy, creativity, clear and effective communication skills, ability to provide constructive and authentic feedback, strategic and visionary thinking, risk taking, positivity, and even confidence. However, description of great leadership skills may overlap with traits and qualities, which once again is how others experience any individual who is in a formal "leadership" position based on professional and/or organizational hierarchy. Whether qualities are innate or learned, leadership skills can be improved and grow with time, experience, and knowledge. There are various opportunities and ways to enhance leadership skills, perhaps best described as self-influenced or internal, versus external or learned from others. Independent activities include reading, writing, and simply seeking opportunities in a serial or simultaneous fashion that involve activities during which one's role and voice influences outcomes. External training for the development of leadership skills

Table 3	
Examples of ways physicians may serve as leaders	
Within the division/ department/hospital	• Service on medical staff committees, i.e., credentials, quality and safety, resuscitation, pharmaceutical, therapeutics, etc. • Oversee division or departmental operational logistics for satellites or specific areas of practice • Program director or associate program director • Create GME wellbeing curriculum for trainees • Coordinate educational curriculum, didactics, for division/ department, and/or community partners • Participate in continuous improvement projects and initiatives for the division/department or other areas of the hospital for which one has passion and professional interest in • Reviewer on the institutional review board and/or other research IRB functions • Grant reviewer
Outside the hospital/ medical center setting	• Local, state, and regional chapters of societies, such as county and state medical societies • Serve on local chapters of various organizations—volunteer on boards of organizations that focus on food insecurity, medical care for uninsured, food banks, blood banks, etc. • Educational speaking engagements for local schools to students, to local and regional school nurses, Early intervention programs, other allied health professionals including speech language pathology and audiology • Represent hospital and institution in collaborative task forces for the community for health care, education, or any topics that improve health • Serve and participate as an advisor for patient support groups
Professional Societies and Specialty	• Program committee member for annual regional and national meetings • Serve as officers for subspecialty societies • Serve on various committees for subspecialty societies and AAO-HNS • Volunteer for ad hoc task force or committees • Serve as reviewer for our peer-reviewed journals • Serve as on editorial board of various journals • Work and support staff for various societies and academy
American Board of Otolaryngology Head and Neck Surgery	• Write questions for subcertification and/or maintenance of certification • Serve as oral board examiners

includes coaching, courses on change management, influence, negotiation, and critically effective communication.

For any physician in a leadership role, if the role is specified in the context of the practice of health care, maintaining practice as a front-line physician provides real-time knowledge and understanding of challenges, and typically supports credibility to other clinicians and clinic staff. Once a physician is in a high administrative leadership role and no longer practices, there may often be challenges with implementing mandated operational strategies under pressure from various factors independent of what clinicians may desire or what may support greatest physician wellbeing. Physicians in a high administrative leadership position may often feel isolated and lonely, unable to share their own true emotions or feelings on a variety of health system changes, decisions, and strategic directions. They may also bear unspoken burden and pressure on behalf of the larger physician body, and/or feel underappreciated by those they lead and serve. Furthermore, highly functioning physicians and surgeons, once reaching such levels of administrative "C-suite" roles, may not always have autonomy that may be expected to be commensurate with his/her "title." One pitfall can be giving up clinical practice all together, losing one's core skills and career in medical/surgical expertise, and sacrificing the professional fulfillment that took decades to train and achieve that is never replaced by anything other than direct patient care.

SUMMARY

Leadership is important in all aspects of a physician's professional life. Choosing to take on a leadership role warrants thoughtful preparation. Leadership skills can be developed with experience, training, coaching, and mentorship. Physicians have an obligation to learn as much as possible about effective leadership so that when an opportunity to lead comes, they will make optimal use of it and feel empowered to contribute to solutions and improvements at all levels of health care. The "best fit" lies in finding the right opportunities for the right reasons at the right time and being prepared to pursue those that will stretch and challenge your professional growth—and do not look back when you do!

DISCLOSURE

The authors have nothing to disclose.

SUGGESTED READINGS

Wei JL. Leadership, engagement, and well being. ENT Today; 2019. Available at: https://www.enttoday.org/article/leadership-engagement-and-well-being/.

Kotter JP. What leaders really do. Harv Bus Rev 1990;68(3):103–11.

Freischlag JA, Silva MM. Bouncing up: resilience and women in academic medicine. J Am Coll Surg 2016;223(2):215–20.

Collins JC. Good to great: why some companies make the leap ... and others don't. New York: HarperBusiness; 2001.

George B, Sims P. True north: discover your authentic leadership. San Francisco (CA): Jossey-Bass/John Wiley & Sons; 2007.

Sinek S. Start with why. Harlow (England): Penguin Books; 2011.

Kibbe MR, Chen H. Leadership in surgery. Switzerland: Springer International; 2016.

Kouzes JM, Posner BZ. The leadership challenge: how to make extraordinary things happen in organizations. Hoboken (NJ): John Wiley & Sons, Inc.; 2017.

Goldsmith M. What got you here won't get you there: how successful people become even more successful. New York: Hyperion; 2007.

"Leadership in Action", SiriuxXM Channel 132, Business Radio Powered by Wharton, Fridays, 9AM-10AM EDT.

Moving Toward Professional Equity in Otolaryngology

Jamie R. Litvack, MD, MS, FARS[a], Robin W. Lindsay, MD[b],*

KEYWORDS

- Equity • Pay equity • Relative value unit • Underrepresented minorities

KEY POINTS

- Prioritization of professional equity is mission critical and should to become a part of institutional and departmental strategy for continued organizational success.
- Professional equity involves pay equity, resources equity, promotion equity, and equitable access to leadership positions.
- Psychologically safety is fundamental to a safe and effective work environment, ensuring that all voices are heard and that some members are not silenced because of fears of retaliation.

INTRODUCTION

Gender-based equity in compensation, access to opportunity and resources, and leadership roles are critical to the health and future of otolaryngology; however, significant gaps continue to persist.[1] Twenty years ago, Dr Linda Brodsky, a professor of otolaryngology, filed suit against Kaleida Health and the State University of New York for pay inequity and retaliation for complaining about this pay inequity.[2] Her case was successfully settled several years later; however, significant gaps in pay, professional opportunities, resource allocation, and leadership roles persist in otolaryngology. Even when women perform the same procedures with the same outcomes and payor mix, women make less.[3–7] Compensation gaps adversely affect workplace culture, work satisfaction and physician well-being, productivity, institutional reputation, recruitment, retention, and quality of care.[8–10] A diverse workforce has been shown to improve outcomes, access to evidenced-based care, and surgical outcomes. In addition, workforce diversity can increase cooperative behaviors that positively impact safety and performance in the operating room (OR).[11–15] All these factors are necessary for organizational success.

Conflict of Interest Statement: No authors have received any funding for this work, or have conflicts of interest.

[a] Department of Medical Education and Clinical Sciences, Elson S. Floyd College of Medicine, Washington State University, Everett, Spokane, Tri-Cities, Vancouver; [b] Department of Otolaryngology – Head & Neck Surgery, Harvard Medical School, Massachusetts Eye and Ear, 243 Charles Street, Boston, MA 02114, USA
* Corresponding author.
E-mail address: Robin_Lindsay@meei.harvard.edu

Otolaryngol Clin N Am 55 (2022) 11–22
https://doi.org/10.1016/j.otc.2021.08.003
0030-6665/22/© 2021 Elsevier Inc. All rights reserved.

oto.theclinics.com

Both the American Medical Association (AMA) and the American Association of Medical Colleges (AAMC) have advocated for policies that promote compensation, transparency, and equity. The AMA, recognizing the negative impact of physician burnout on patient care, added physician wellness as a fourth major goal for the organization, with equal weight to improving patient care, lowering cost, and improving outcomes.[16,17] The AAMC issued a call to action on gender equity in 2020, acknowledging equity as a key factor in achieving excellence in medicine.[18,19] So why, despite a wealth of data demonstrating the negative impact of compensation gaps,[20] does otolaryngology continue to have one of the largest gender pay gaps in health care[21–23]?

To discuss professional equity, it is important to understand the important differences in meaning between equality and equity. Equality means that everyone receives the same treatment and support, whereas equity means that everyone receives equal opportunity to achieve success by getting the support they need to thrive and succeed.[24] Gender pay gap is the difference between the amount of money paid to women and men performing the same or similar job with similar levels of experience.[21] For example, pay can be unequal but still be equitable if the work that is being performed is not comparable. In contrast, pay inequity is the notion that an individual's pay is unfair or not equal to someone else performing a similar job with the same level of experience and productivity. Defining what constitutes comparable work in a fair and transparent manner is an important step to ensuring pay equity. Both pay equity and the equitable distribution of resources and opportunities that allow surgeons to be productive are 2 elements critical to achieving professional equity.

In this article, we review the literature illustrating the severity of the gender-based gap among working otolaryngologists. We then make recommendations for areas of improvement and strategies for achieving professional equity based on objective data. Although we primarily focus on gender-based disparities in this article, we believe professional equity regardless of age, race, color, religion, national origin, sexual orientation, and gender identity is critical to clinical excellence, innovation and the future of our field.

Scope of the Problem

Compensation gaps in otolaryngology exist based on multiple factors including gender, race and ethnicity, and subspeciality, depending on the institutional and departmental compensation plans. According to the 2019 AAMC report "Promising Practices," female otolaryngologists are paid 77 cents on the dollar compared with their male colleagues.[21] Even after accounting for age, experience, faculty rank, research productivity, and clinical revenue, significant gender pay gaps exist across all levels of academic seniority[5,6,25] and can be seen at the time of first hiring.[26] In addition, the intersectionality of race and gender exacerbates pay inequity for women of color.[27,28] The AAMC has 2 new initiatives to address the status of women of color in academic medicine: the Women of Color Intersectionality Working Group and the Women of Color Data Site. Pay gaps widen with age despite controlling for multiple factors,[29] and this observation is accentuated in fields with greater educational requirements and a lower percentage of women or underrepresented minorities (URM) in the field.[1]

Significant pay gaps for the same amount of work performed can exist between and within subspecialities depending on institutional and departmental compensation plans or payor mix. Relative value units (RVUs) can introduce significant disparities between otolaryngology subspecialties when RVUs do not appropriately reflect the total work performed or the actual revenue generated for a specific procedure.[30,31] There is also evidence of gender bias in the valuation of wRVUs for specific procedures.[32,33] Otolaryngology compensation plans should align with departmental goals and values and be designed to incentivize high-quality care to all patients. These plans should also support necessary non-revenue-generating administrative and research activities that provide value to a department and improve institutional reputation, such as education (mentorship and training), patient care, and provider wellness. Compensation plans should value the clinical contributions of all faculty members, recognizing the bias of RVU-only and cash-only systems, and maintain provider accountability for appropriate documentation, billing, resource utilization, and the delivery of high-quality care.[25]

Otolaryngology has a successful recent track record of attracting women with 36% of otolaryngology residents being female.[34,35] However, only 17% of otolaryngologists are female[36] and only 3.5% to 5.1% of department chairs are women.[35,37] Achieving not only a seat at the table for women and URM, but a voice on committees that determine institutional and departmental compensation plans, is a vital step toward achieving professional equity.

Achieving professional equity regardless of race or gender once individuals have entered the pipeline will be the focus of this article. The first step to achieving professional equity in otolaryngology is leadership prioritization of equity as mission critical. Other vital steps will include improving organizational culture, developing systems for advocacy, understanding what constitutes equal pay in otolaryngology, developing transparent and reoccurring equity review processes,[38] and promoting women into leadership positions.[18,20]

Prioritization of professional equity as mission critical

Prioritization of professional equity by local and national leadership is vital to achieving compensation equity. Some specialties have reacted aggressively and made affirmative strides toward achieving professional equity. After the publication of the AAMC report "Promising Practices"[21] in which the gender pay gap in cardiology was determined to be 78 cents on the dollar, the American College of Cardiology (ACC) almost immediately started on the "2019 ACC Health Policy Statement on Cardiologist Compensation and Opportunity Equity." The ACC recognized that compensation and access to opportunity and resources are critical to the health and future of their workforce.[10] Leadership at other academic and health care institutions, such as MIT and Medical College of Wisconsin, have responded similarly by creating systems for correcting inequities once they were discovered.[39] The AAMC has put forth best practices to move toward compensation equity in health care and highlights institutions that have prioritized professional equity.[21]

The AMA has also taken a lead in this arena by advocating for a multitiered approach:

- Developing institutional and departmental policies that promote transparency in defining initial and subsequent physician compensation.
- Promoting equal base pay based on objective criteria.
- Working to promote training for individuals in positions to decide physician compensation on the topics of implicit bias and compensation determination.
- Encouraging an approach that prioritizes the identification of gender disparity, along with the oversight of compensation models, metrics, and actual total compensation for all employed physicians.
- Urging institutions and organizations to begin educational programs to help all physicians negotiate equitable compensation.

Professional equity *must* become a priority for otolaryngology. Institutions that are doing this well should be encouraged to publicize their practices.[18] Organizations should identify their organizational mission, goals, and values and then align compensation with these goals and values.[10,19,21] A first step is to make professional equity an explicit part of the mission statement of national organizations, institutions, and departments. Prioritization of professional equity should include compensation, resource, promotion, and leadership equity.

Organization culture and advocacy

A positive workplace culture, where faculty feel a sense of belonging,[40] has been shown to improve both faculty quality of life, patient care, and the financial health of an organization.[3,7,21] Our historical culture has often fallen short of this goal, where 41% of female otolaryngologists report experiencing some form of harassment.[41] Microaggressions, microinsults, assaults, invalidations, unconscious/conscious bias, and power abuse limit a person's ability to thrive in their work environment and are common barriers to a positive organizational culture.[24] Leaders must remove the culture that women and URMs are to blame for their compensation inequities because of poor negotiation skills, poor coding, working less, and having children, because pay gaps have been proven to exist when controlling for these factors.[35,42] The AAMC Statement on Gender Equities puts forth the mandate that the distorted cultural narratives in academic medicine that insist that "women work less" must end.[43] The 2019 report "Women in the Workplace" by McKinsey and Co recommends holding senior leadership accountable for equity and diversity concerns,[44] because holding leaders accountable for moving their organizations from intention to impact can be a critical game changer.[45]

Understanding that professional equity concerns are erosive to organizational cultures, some institutions, such as Brigham and Women's Hospital (BWH), have started Professionalism Committees and developed systems to identify and act on areas of concerns in their community. Building a Professionalism Committee involves including representation from diverse stakeholders including human resources (HR), clinical faculty, and hospital leadership. Through thoughtful and iterative process mapping, the team at BWH developed multiple reporting mechanisms, including in person, electronic, and by phone. To combat the historically negative perception that faculty have for HR, BWH worked to create an improved relationship between HR and faculty by adding a senior HR individual directly responsible for faculty. They also used the skills of the HR department to help to investigate faculty concerns, using the HR staff as trained investigators. When disputes arise, the goal is for HR to partner with departmental leadership and to provide support both for the individual filing the complaint and the subject of the complaint; they have created documents and provided education to departmental leadership on how to document concerning behavior so that there is a record of reoccurring behaviors independent of leadership changes. In addition, mental health, coaching, and mediation support services are provided for both sides. Realizing the importance of leadership that prioritizes positive organizational culture and professional equity, they have also revised the search process for department chairs and division directors.

Although the initial efforts of the Professionalism Committee identified individuals erosive to organizational culture, advanced efforts have identified "hot spots" within departments or specific work areas. Identification of these "hot spots" (by careful monitoring and mapping out the experience of retaliation and professional equity concerns) has allowed them to start to operationalize systems to improve behaviors that would have otherwise been difficult to detect. The goal is to change organizational culture, including the expectation that retaliation and professional inequities will not be tolerated, so that at some point the committee will no longer be needed.

Moving from a mandate for equity to changing systems requires understanding where there are true problems, so that targeted solutions can be developed. The obstacles to equity may be different for individual departments and divisions within an institution. Dr Jennifer Shin, the Vice Chair of Academic Affairs for Otolaryngology at BWH, has worked with the department of surgery leadership at BWH to develop departmental surveys guided by information obtained through focus groups and one-on-one conversations with stake holders within the department and institution. This collaboration has helped determine high-priority items and concerns and led directly to program development. One of the first action items was addressing child care needs during the pandemic. This type of survey and program development could be used by departments and institutions to focus on the topic of professional equity. An important part of survey usage is a commitment from leadership that action will be taken to correct system errors discovered by the survey. Other strategies include the development of a tool box for leadership to guide development of an annual review process using best practices, unconscious bias training, a clear system of reporting equity and work environment concerns, and making sure leaders are accountable for equity goals.

Defining equal work in otolaryngology creating systems to ensure equal pay for equal work

Defining equal work. Defining equal work in otolaryngology will, in part, depend on organizational goals and values and is made more challenging by the complicated reimbursement structures that exist in health care.[21] Both revenue-generating and non-revenue-generating clinical, research, and administrative activities must be considered. Some departments may also prioritize teaching and community service. With regard to clinical revenue, consideration should be made for differences in RVU generation, reimbursement, and downstream revenue between subspecialties. Many different compensation plans are used currently: RVU-only models, cash-based models, salaried models, and mixed X + Y + Z models, each with their own benefits and pitfalls. The chosen model may need to be different for individual departments. Nevertheless, the goal should be to prioritize equity, to make individuals feel valued for their individual contributions to the department, and thereby drive performance and high-quality patient care to all patients.

Relative value units-only systems. We submit that RVU-only systems for otolaryngology have the greatest risk of creating significant pay gaps and can potentially negatively impact billing behavior. There is evidence to suggest that current work RVUs are misvalued[31] because changes in work RVUs have not reflected changes in technology in some specialties and because work RVUs may continue to undervalue cognitive effort. Addressing the misevaluations in work RVUs so that the values reflect true differences in time and intensity could further reduce disparities in physician compensation.[30] The variation in work RVUs across health care specialties stems from 3 sources: the number of hours physicians work per year, the ability of certain specialties to generate more RVUs per hour worked than specialties that rely on face-to-face office visits, and misvalued work RVUs.[30,31] Gender bias exists and persists for women's health as well. Analysis using 2015 CPT data showed that 72% of male urologic procedures had higher work RVUs and total RVUs than equivalent female gynecologic procedures.[32,33] Total fee and reimbursement was higher in 84%. On average, urologic procedures reimbursed 28% higher than gynecologic equivalents.

RVU-only compensation models are particularly problematic for otolaryngology because of the diversity of procedures performed by different subspecialties within otolaryngology. The RVU system is now a 30-year-old system and undervalues many of the procedures performed in specific subspecialities in otolaryngology, creating a system in which some subspecialities can bill significantly more RVUs than others in the same amount of OR time. Making an RVU-only system even more problematic is that despite higher RVU potential per OR day, those procedures can generate less revenue per RVU compared with others because of lower reimbursement rates secondary to payor mix in some practices. Compensation plans that depend only on RVUs undervalue high-revenue-generating clinical care including cash practices, international care, favorable payor mix, procedures requiring a high level of expertise but with low work RVUs, and time. Furthermore, RVU-only systems run the risks of misaligning accountability and compensation, thereby incentivizing high RVU procedures; this can result in providers avoiding low RVU procedures and consequently reduce the availability for patient care. Furthermore, some RVU-only compensation models pay providers based on RVUs submitted and not RVUs reimbursed, incentivizing over coding of RVUs without ensuring appropriate precertification and documentation to ensure reimbursement of the submitted RVUs. Overcoding and undercoding can lead to systems errors that negatively impact both colleagues and the quality and cost of care that we deliver to patients.[46]

Nationally, the AAO-HNS can wield their influence to promote the coverage and valuation of specific codes, so that patients can receive needed care, and the codes are a better reflection of the time, effort, and expertise for the work required. Regarding inappropriately valued RVUs, the membership of the AAO-HNS should make the appropriate committee chairs aware of RVU discrepancies so that the subspeciality chairs can work with the 3 P committee on whether or not revaluation is needed for currently undervalued codes or if a new code is needed for a new procedure. Similarly, if there are codes that are repeatedly denied because of lack of coverage in specific plans, or if the insurance company's accepted indications no longer represent the current standard of care, work can be done at the academy level to align coverage with the standard of care.

Locally, faculty should be educated about their federal and state rights for compensation equity and what to do when they feel that their compensation is not equitable. Faculty should be educated about the compensation plan in their department and how the department receives funds from the institution. Courses on negotiation, unconscious bias, and coding can also be considered.

Salaried systems. The Veterans Affairs (VA) and Mayo health care systems are 2 of the most well-known salaried systems. Several features of the VA medical system contribute to the reduction and/or absence of a gender-based pay gap across otolaryngology and other surgical subspecialities.[47] Objective criteria are used to establish pay. Pay is transparent and publicly available. Starting salaries for new hires are similar for men and women surgeons. Stepwise increases, recurring systematic reviews (including biennial market pay reviews), and retroactive adjustments for missed or delayed reviews contribute to a sense of fairness and pay equity. Salaried systems do have the benefit of transparency but may not be equitable if promotion and resource allocation are not equitable. A study from the Mayo Clinic, which has used a structured salary-only compensation model for decades, reports gender, race, and ethnicity pay equity in 96% of cases; however, men had twice as many compensable leadership roles and more protected time.[48] Leveling and inequities in promotion and leadership can cause profound pay inequities that are not identified when only analyzing pay based on position. Furthermore, productivity, resource equity, protected research time, and quality of care should also be considered for a system to truly be equitable.

Faculty accountability and education: cost containment, billing, professionalism, patient outcomes, research, and administrative tasks. An ideal compensation system would include accountability for cost containment, appropriate billing, professionalism, and patient outcomes to incentivize a positive organizational culture and high-quality care. Accountability for cost containment and appropriate billing leads to financial strength of the department/organization. Emphasis should be placed on the importance of cost containment, so that faculty treat clinics and the ORs as if they were the one paying the overhead; this is particularly important in academic practices, because the overhead costs are often underrecognized by providers, or at least are not tied to personal compensation.

Referral sources, hours worked, procedure duration, complexity of patients, and clinical efficiency can all impact productivity and reimbursement. Referral sources and practices should be evaluated for equitable access to a diverse patient population. Even when women work the same hours and have the same surgical times with the same outcomes, they make less.[5,49,50] Limitations in referral networks can also be responsible for female surgeons working under their level of training.[51,52] In addition, gender homophily in a surgical faculty network has been demonstrated to impede female career advancement among academic surgeons, pointing to the need for improved networking systems for junior and senior female faculty.[53]

Consideration should also be made to the use of outcomes utilization such as PROM instruments or other objective measures to quantify outcomes, a practice already adopted by many surgical subspecialties. The passage of the Medicare Access and CHIP Reauthorization Act in 2015, which created the Quality Payment Programs, laid out the pathway for promoting quality- or value-based reimbursement, beginning with 2017 as the first year of gathering benchmark data and impacting compensation starting in 2019.

Efficiency is another consideration. There may be value to analyzing differences in efficiencies among physicians, including the complexity of care, visit duration, quality of care, and support staff and room utilization. However, if one provider sees twice as many patients with the same resources and outcomes when compared with another provider, then equal compensation is not equitable. These individual differences need to be understood so that clinical support can be provided that results in the maximum efficiency and quality of each provider.

Compensation plans also need to determine how non-revenue-generating tasks, such as innovation, unfunded research, teaching, and administrative tasks, are supported by the department. Women are often assigned to uncompensated but time-consuming administrative roles that have been referred to as "institutional housekeeping," which do not lead to promotion but are vital to the organization.[54]

Organizations should prioritize developing a fair and transparent metric-driven annual review process for professional equity based on clear organizational goals.[38,55] Systems designed for equity review should be transparent, metric driven, and should appropriately incentivize surgeons in alignment with organizational goals. Additionally, they should be able to identify outliers, have external unbiased oversight, promote leadership, and uphold provider accountability. Gaps and outliers that are identified should be corrected or justified by departmental leadership to build and grow trust within the system. Finally, they should provide a system for advocacy to prevent retaliation and address compensation concerns when they arise. Reviews should be performed at least annually and with each new hire.

Create systems to ensure equal access to opportunity and resources

Equity of opportunity in terms of resources, achievements, and positions should be a priority for departments and institutions. In addition, factors that impact compensation for otolaryngologists within our community should be identified to allow for a framework for comparable work/equity review evaluation. The factors that make faculty successful may vary by the individual and by the specialty; this may depend on personal workflow preferences and the specific subspecialty needs. Equity means ensuring that individuals have the resources that they need to succeed. Factors that can impact productivity for otolaryngologists include support staff availability, alignment of support staff cost with the support received, OR block time allocation, office space, clinic room allocation, overhead cost, and referral management. In addition, there should be open discussion within the group about other factors that individuals feel impact productivity.[3]

Leadership and promotion

The lack of women in leadership positions in otolaryngology creates extreme power differentials in our field. This power differential places men in the position to prioritize gender equity or not.[56] Because only 3.5% of otolaryngology department chairs are women, male sponsorship is vital to achieving professional equity in our field.[35] Because organizational and professional networks are important for promotion and advancement, and because gender homophily exists,[53] women are at a disadvantage when leadership opportunities arise. Sponsorship from senior male leaders is critical to reducing the career advancement gap. We need to continue to build a diverse workforce including not only recruitment of female and URM into otolaryngology residency programs but also sponsorship of women and URM into meaningful leadership positions and committees within our organizations. Sponsorship, elevating with intention, and understanding and acknowledging the factors that perpetuate inequities will help to close the gender gap.

The importance of having male sponsorship and mentorship is highlighted in the book "Athena Rising," and much has been written on how men can support female physicians.[18,57] A 2014 gender parity study demonstrated that 50% of women entering the work force have their eye on the C-suite but in just 2 years this number drops by 60% not because of parental or marital status but because of the lack of meaningful recognition and support from their managers necessary to support career advancement. The recruitment process of senior leadership positions should include at least 2 women candidates. This recommendation is based on the finding of a 2016 Harvard Business Review article, which demonstrated that if there is only 1 woman in your candidate pool, then statistically there is 0 chance that she will be hired.[58] However, if 2 of 4 candidates are female, there is 50% likelihood that a female will be hired. Research has demonstrated that women stay in roles longer and are promoted to lower roles when compared with male colleagues.[35] However, equal number of female and male faculty reported working part-time.[35] Tracking of hiring and promotions data will help to identify these problems within specific organizations.

A commitment of those in power to create real change is a critical early step,[18] but understanding the negative impact of gender bias and developing a systematic approach to eliminating the biased decision making that perpetuates inequities in the workplace is needed.[51,59] Correction of workplace discrimination requires more than implicit bias training alone; it requires an understanding of common gender stereotypes and how these stereotypes negatively impact females in the workplace.[51] Female surgeons report gender bias in the workplace as a major cause of burnout.[60] Women are more likely to volunteer for activities that will not advance their careers because they are fearful of the repercussions that they will face if they do not do the extra work; this often delays promotion because the activities that they are doing are not valued by promotion committees. Women are subject to significant gender backlash when they advocate on their own behalf.[44,61] Women may not negotiate at work, not because they lack negotiation skills but because they understand the negative ramifications when they do.[61,62] Women often find themselves in a double bind and an "impression management dilemma" when they are interested in leadership.[63] Men can be seen as both warm and competent, whereas women are either seen as warm and incompetent or competent and cold. Tokenism can worsen the work environment for women, because they can be seen as not worthy of their appointed role and worsen organizational culture. Senior leaders should articulate new social norms, publicly stating that women should advocate on their own behalf and then ensure that there are not negative consequences for this behavior so that these norms permeate through the organization and become the new normal.[56]

SUMMARY

Progress has been made in otolaryngology. However, much is left to do to achieve professional gender equity. We have a growing female talent pool,[64] and we need to manage our talent appropriately to ensure the future success of our field. Professional equity in otolaryngology will be achieved by leadership prioritization of equity as mission critical, understanding what constitutes equal pay in otolaryngology, developing transparent and recurring equity review processes, promoting women into leadership positions, and understanding and acknowledging the factors that perpetuate inequities. Sponsorship of women and increasing the number of women in leadership is important to attract and retain top talent, to ensure high-value care to all patients, and to create organizational climate that inspires excellent patient care and promotes provider well-being. The best way forward is one based on trust, transparency, inclusion, and identification of best practices that are currently being used successfully.

REFERENCES

1. Adamy, Overberg. Women in elite jobs face stubborn pay gap. Wall Street J. Available at: https://www.wsj.com/articles/women-in-elite-jobs-face-stubborn-pay-gap-1463502938. Accessed April, 2021.
2. Avery-Washington E. Court case: Brodsky v. Kaleida Health and State University of New York at Buffalo. AAUW; 2008. Available at: https://ww3.aauw.org/resource/brodsky-v-kaleida-health-and-state-university-of-new-york-at-buffalo. Accessed June 19, 2021.
3. Jena AB, Olenski AR, Blumenthal DM. Sex differences in physician salary in US Public Medical Schools. JAMA Intern Med 2016;176(9):1294–304.
4. Seabury SA, Chandra A, Jena AB. Trends in the earnings of male and female health care professionals in the United States, 1987 to 2010. JAMA Intern Med 2013;173(18):1748–50.
5. Sharoky CE, Sellers MM, Keele LJ, et al. Does surgeon sex matter?: practice patterns and outcomes of female and male surgeons. Ann Surg 2018;267(6):1069–76.
6. Chandrasekhar S. Women in otolaryngology: do we belong here? ENTtoday; 2018. Available at: https://www.enttoday.org/article/women-in-otolaryngology-do-we-belong-here/.
7. Jagsi R, Griffith KA, Stewart A, et al. Gender differences in the salaries of physician researchers. JAMA 2012;307(22):2410–7.
8. Physicians adopt plan to combat pay gap in medicine. Chicago: AMA; 2018. Accessed April 2021.
9. Lewis SJ, Mehta LS, Douglas PS, et al. Changes in the professional lives of cardiologists over 2 decades. J Am Coll Cardiol 2017;69(4):452–62.
10. Douglas PS, Biga C, Burns KM, et al. 2019 ACC health policy statement on cardiologist compensation and opportunity equity. J Am Coll Cardiol 2019;74(15):1947–65.

11. Tsugawa Y, Jena AB, Figueroa JF, et al. Comparison of hospital mortality and re-admission rates for medicare patients treated by male vs female physicians. JAMA Intern Med 2017;177(2):206–13.
12. Dwyer S, Richard OC, Chadwick K. Gender diversity in management and firm performance: the influence of growth orientation and organizational culture. J Business Res 2003;56(12):1009–19.
13. Wallis CJ, Ravi B, Coburn N, et al. Comparison of postoperative outcomes among patients treated by male and female surgeons: a population based matched cohort study. BMJ 2017;359:j4366.
14. Berthold HK, Gouni-Berthold I, Bestehorn KP, et al. Physician gender is associated with the quality of type 2 diabetes care. J Intern Med 2008;264(4):340–50.
15. Myers C, Sutcliffe K. How discrimination against female doctors hurts patients. Harvard business review; 2021. Available at: https://hbr.org/2018/08/how-discrimination-against-female-doctors-hurts-patients. Accessed June 5, 2021.
16. Bodenheimer T, Sinsky C. From triple to quadruple aim: care of the patient requires care of the provider. Ann Fam Med 2014;12(6):573–6.
17. Aparicio A, Sinsky CA, Lim B, et al. Creating the organizational foundation for joy in medicine. Chicago: Professional Statement from AMA; 2018.
18. Acosta DA, Lautenberger DM, Castillo-Page L, et al. Achieving gender equity is our responsibility: leadership matters. Acad Med 2020;95(10):1468–71.
19. Aamc statement on gender equity. 2020. Available at: https://www.aamc.org/system/files/2020-01/AAMC%20Gender%20Equity%20Statement_0.pdf. Accessed April 1, 2021.
20. Heisler CA, Miller P, Stephens EH, et al. Leading from Behind: Paucity of gender equity statements and policies among professional surgical societies. Am J Surg 2020;220(5):1132–5.
21. Dandar V, Lautenberger D, Garrison G. Promising practices for understanding and addressing salary equity at U.S. Medical schools. A report of the association of American Medical Colleges. 2019. Available at: https://store.aamc.org/downloadable/download/sample/sample_id/278/. Accessed April 1, 2021.
22. Doximity. 2020 physician compensation report. 2021. Available at: https://www.doximity.com/2020_compensation_report. Accessed June 2021.
23. Lindsay R. Gender-based pay discrimination in otolaryngology. Laryngoscope 2021;131(5):989–95.
24. DIB and E Toolkit, Harvard Human Resources Center for Workplace Advancement 2020; Cambridge(MA).
25. Sanfey H, Crandall M, Shaughnessy E, et al. Strategies for identifying and closing the gender salary gap in surgery. J Am Coll Surg Aug 2017;225(2):333–8.
26. Lo Sasso AT, Richards MR, Chou C-F, et al. The $16,819 pay gap for newly trained physicians: the unexplained trend of men earning more than women. Health Aff 2011;30(2):193–201.
27. Miller K, Vagins D. The simple truth about the gender paygap: 2019 update from the AAUW. 2019. Available at: https://wwwaauworg/app/uploads/2020/02/Simple-Truth-Update-2019_v2-002pdf. Accessed April 1, 2021.
28. Usual weekly earnings of wage and salary workers. Fourth quarter 2018. 2019. Available at: https://www.bls.gov/bls/news-release/wkyeng.htm. Accessed January 17, 2019.
29. Butkus R, Serchen J, Moyer DV, et al. Achieving gender equity in physician compensation and career advancement: a position paper of the American College of Physicians. Ann Intern Med 2018;168(10):721–3.

30. Marks K, Das S, Brandt C, et al. Analysis of disparities in physician compensation. 2019. Available at: http://www.medpac.gov/docs/default-source/contractor-reports/jan19_medpac_disparities_physiciancompensationreport_cvr_contractor_sec.pdf. Accessed June 2021.

31. Zuckerman S, Berenson RA, Lallemand NC, et al. Realign physician payment incentives in Medicare to achieve payment equity among specialties, expand the supply of primary care physicians, and improve the value of care for beneficiaries. 2015. Available at: http://webarchive.urban.org/UploadedPDF/2000059-Realign-Physician-Payment-Incentives-in-Medicare.pdf. Accessed April 1, 2021.

32. Goff BA, Muntz HG, Cain JM. Comparison of 1997 Medicare relative value units for gender-specific procedures: is Adam still worth more than eve? Gynecol Oncol 1997;66(2):313–9.

33. Benoit MF, Ma JF, Upperman BA. Comparison of 2015 Medicare relative value units for gender-specific procedures: Gynecologic and gynecologic-oncologic versus urologic CPT coding. Has time healed gender-worth? Gynecol Oncol 2017;144(2):336–42.

34. The majority of U.S. medical students are women, new data show. AAMC; 2019. Available at: https://www.aamc.org/news-insights/press-releases/%20majority-us-medical-students-are-women-new-data-show. Accessed June 2020.

35. Diana M, Lautenberger M, Valerie M, Dandar M. 2018-2019 the state of women in academic medicine: exploring pathways to equity. 2020. Available at: https://www.aamc.org/data-reports/data/2018-2019-state-women-academic-medicine-exploring-pathways-equity. Accessed April 1, 2021.

36. Active physicians by sex and specialty. 2017. Available at: https://www.aamc.org/data-reports/workforce/%20interactive-data/active-physicians-sex-and-specialty-2017. Accessed June 2020.

37. Epperson M, Gouveia CJ, Tabangin ME, et al. Female representation in otolaryngology leadership roles. Laryngoscope 2020;130(7):1664–9.

38. Morris M, Chen H, Heslin MJ, et al. A structured compensation plan improves but does not erase the sex pay gap in surgery. Ann Surg 2018;268(3):442–8.

39. Closing the gender pay gap in medicine: a roadmap for healthcare organizations and the women physicians who work for them. Chicago: Springer; 2021.

40. McPeek-Hinz E, Boazak M, Sexton JB, et al. Clinician burnout associated with sex, clinician type, work culture, and use of electronic health records. JAMA Netw Open 2021;4(4):e215686.

41. Lawlor C, Kawai K, Tracy L, et al. Women in otolaryngology: experiences of being female in the specialty. Laryngoscope 2020.

42. Cochran A, Neumayer LA, Elder WB. Barriers to careers identified by women in academic surgery: a grounded theory model. Am J Surg 2019;218(4):780–5.

43. Bohnet I. What works: gender equality. The Belknap Press of Harvard University Press; 2016.

44. McKinsey. Women in the workplace report. San Francisco(CA): McKinsey and Company; 2019.

45. Irde S. The Growing Importance of Creating an Inclusive Workplace. Catalyst India WRC. 2016. Available at: https://www.td.org/insights/the-growing-importance-of-creating-an-inclusive-workplace. Accessed April 1, 2021.

46. Gawande A. The cost Conundrum. Chicago: The New Yorker; 2009.

47. Dermody SM, Litvack JR, Randall JA, et al. Compensation of otolaryngologists in the Veterans health administration: is there a gender gap? Laryngoscope 2019;129(1):113–8.

48. Hayes SN, Noseworthy JH, Farrugia G. A structured compensation plan results in equitable physician compensation: a single-center analysis. Chicago: Elsevier; 2020. p. 35–43.
49. Dossa F, Baxter NN. Reducing gender bias in surgery. Br J Surg 2018;105(13): 1707–9.
50. Dossa F, Simpson AN, Sutradhar R, et al. Sex-based disparities in the hourly earnings of surgeons in the fee-for-service system in Ontario, Canada. JAMA Surg 2019;154(12):1134–42.
51. Hutchison K. Four types of gender bias affecting women surgeons and their cumulative impact. J Med Ethics 2020;46(4):236–41.
52. Zeltzer D. Gender homophily in referral networks: Consequences for the medicare physician earnings gap. Am Econ J Appl Econ 2020;12(2):169–97.
53. Suurna MV, Leibbrandt A. Underrepresented women leaders: lasting impact of gender homophily in surgical faculty networks. Laryngoscope 2021. https://doi.org/10.1002/lary.29681.
54. Zhuge Y, Kaufman J, Simeone DM, et al. Is there still a glass ceiling for women in academic surgery? Ann Surg 2011;253(4):637–43.
55. Beebe KS, Krell ES, Rynecki ND, et al. The effect of sex on orthopaedic surgeon income. J Bone Joint Surg Am 2019;101(17):e87.
56. Chang E, Milkman KL. Improving decisions that affect gender equality in the workplace. Chicago: Organizational Dynamics; 2020. p. 49.
57. Sinha M. 10 ways to support female physicians. In: Presentation to the Massachusetts Medical Society. 2018.
58. Johnson SK, Hekman DR, Chan ET. If there's only one woman in your candidate pool, there's statistically no chance she'll be hired. Chicago: Harvard Business Review; 2016.
59. Begeny CT, Ryan MK, Moss-Racusin CA, et al. In some professions, women have become well represented, yet gender bias persists—Perpetuated by those who think it is not happening. Sci Adv 2020;6(26):eaba7814.
60. Lu PW, Columbus AB, Fields AC, et al. Gender differences in surgeon burnout and barriers to career satisfaction: a qualitative exploration. J Surg Res 2020; 247:28–33.
61. Artz B, Goodall A, Oswald A. Research: women ask for raises as often as men, but are less likely to get them. Harvard Business Review; 2018. Available at: https://hbr.org/2018/06/research-women-ask-for-raises-as-often-as-men-but-are-less-likely-to-get-them. Accessed April 1, 2021.
62. Amanatullah ET, Morris MW. Negotiating gender roles: Gender differences in assertive negotiating are mediated by women's fear of backlash and attenuated when negotiating on behalf of others. J Personal Soc Psychol 2010;98(2):256.
63. Rudman LA, Phelan JE. Backlash effects for disconfirming gender stereotypes in organizations. Res Organ Behav 2008;28:61–79.
64. Linscheid LJ, Holliday EB, Ahmed A, et al. Women in academic surgery over the last four decades. PLoS One 2020;15(12):e0243308.

Finding the Right Job
Locum Tenens and Private Practice

Samantha J. Hauff, MD[a],*, D. Scott Fortune, MD[b]

KEYWORDS

- Locum tenens • Otolaryngology careers • Travel

KEY POINTS

- Locum tenens otolaryngology is a career choice that offers flexibility and variety.
- There are several practical and lifestyle considerations when choosing a locums assignment.
- Negotiation is key when working with a locum tenens agency.
- The locum tenens physician is an independent contractor and has to furnish her own benefits.

FINDING THE RIGHT JOB IN OTOLARYNGOLOGY: LOCUM TENENS

Samantha J. Hauff, MD.
  Locum Tenens 2017–2018.
  Private Practice 2019–present.

Introduction

In a rapidly changing health care environment with an ever-increasing array of practice models, selecting the career path that is the best fit for one's professional goals and lifestyle is a daunting task. There is little formal education about the pros and cons of different practice settings or reimbursement structures. Most residents on the verge of graduating know little other than what they have been exposed to during training, which is typically academic and/or hospital-employed otolaryngology. However, the reality is that more than half of otolaryngologists are in some form of private practice,[1] and it is important to consider the full spread of career options if one wants to find the one that will provide her with the highest job satisfaction while also balancing other aspects of life.

[a] Sunset ENT, 4282 Genesee Avenue, Suite 202, San Diego, CA 92117, USA; [b] Allergy & ENT Associates of Middle TN, PC, 3901 Central Pike Suite 351, Hermitage, TN 37076, USA
* Corresponding author.
E-mail address: sunsetentsd@gmail.com

Otolaryngol Clin N Am 55 (2022) 23–31
https://doi.org/10.1016/j.otc.2021.07.007
0030-6665/22/© 2021 Elsevier Inc. All rights reserved.

oto.theclinics.com

Some important questions to ask oneself when deciding on a potential practice model:

- How important is it for me to have control over my schedule, choice of electronic health records (EHR), equipment purchasing, and day-to-day minutiae?
- Do I want to understand and/or manage the business side of my practice?
- Do I want to have someone who is considered my "boss," whether it be a department chair, clinic manager, or practice owner?
- How often do I want to be on call, whether it be for my patients alone or for an entire practice or a hospital (or 3)?
- Am I someone who is driven by productivity incentives, or will that just create unnecessary stress in my life?

For some otolaryngologists, the answers to these questions are unclear, especially for those who have never before practiced outside of residency. For those who feel that they need more exposure to different practice models before they can decide which is right for them, locum tenens may offer a great opportunity to test the proverbial waters. There is no better way to figure out the perks, pitfalls, and personalities of a practice than to immerse oneself in it for a few weeks or months at a time. For other otolaryngologists, locums may offer a financial bridge when between jobs or when life circumstances preclude a longer-term commitment, and for some older otolaryngologists, locum tenens' work may provide a change of pace as they transition to retirement.

Background

Locum tenens is Latin for "place holder." The concept of a locum tenens ("locums") physician originated in the late 1970s as a way of managing burnout among rural physicians. The University of Utah and the Robert Wood Johnson Foundation joined forces to create a network of physicians that could cover for rural practices when their owners needed time off for continuing medical education, vacation, or sick days.[2,3] Today, locum tenens is a billion-dollar industry, with physicians working all across the country, in rural, suburban, and urban settings alike.[2] In 2001, the North American Locum Tenens Organization (NALTO) was formed within the industry to help set and maintain professional and legal standards. NALTO's Website currently lists 85 member agencies.

Most locums jobs are for temporary positions where a practice or a hospital has a physician out on leave or needs more help handling patient volume on an intermittent basis. Some, though, are looking to hire someone temporarily with the goal of eventually filling a permanent position. A search of 2 of the largest locums agencies, CompHealth and LocumTenens.com, reveal 69 and 276 active listings, respectively, with listings in nearly every state. Job descriptions range from call coverage only to part-time clinic only, with everything in between. According to NALTO, an estimated three-quarters of all hospitals use locum tenens physicians.[4]

Quality of Care in Locum Tenens

It is only natural to wonder if augmenting a hospital's or a clinic's permanent medical staff with "place holders" would result in wavering quality of care or poorer patient outcomes. Given that primary care and general surgery are 2 of the specialties that use locums physicians most frequently, the available data largely reflect data gathered from these specialists. A retrospective cohort study of more than 1.8 million Medicare beneficiaries hospitalized between 2009 and 2014 showed no significant difference in 30-day mortality between those patients treated by locum tenens physicians versus those treated by nonlocum tenens physicians.[5] A study of more than 112,000 Medicare beneficiaries who underwent common neurosurgical procedures by either locum tenens or permanent staff neurosurgeons found no significant difference in complication rates, length of hospitalization, or costs.[6] In a survey of members of the American Pediatric Surgical Association, 64% of respondents believed that surgical care in a locum tenens situation was inferior to that provided by a permanent community-based pediatric surgeon. However, most of the respondents (87%) supported the use of locums physicians for short-term coverage.[7]

Financial and Medicolegal Considerations

One of the appeals of locums work is that the average daily reimbursement is typically more than one would earn in a day of work at a long-term position. Hospitals pay a premium for the locum tenens agency's services—it is estimated that a locums physician costs the employer 25% to 30% more than a permanent staff would cost.[8] For most positions, the locums company will assist with expedited licensing and credentialing, and all costs associated with this are usually covered, although some posts specifically state you must already have a state medical license. The agency will also arrange all travel, lodging, and transportation needs. A standard hotel room is usually offered, although it is possible to negotiate other arrangements, such as a short-term vacation rental or an executive apartment.

With regard to compensation, typical offers start with a daily rate that varies depending on the agency, the hospital, the location, and the job demands. This initial offered amount is only a portion of what the hospital is paying to the locum tenens agency, so there is typically room for negotiation. When selecting an assignment and negotiating pay, be aware of what comprises a work "day," as this could range from an 8-hour clinic day to 24 hours of call coverage. In many cases, an hourly overtime rate is also negotiated, and it is certainly nice to be paid for your time if you spend an additional hour or two charting at the end of a clinic day.

Locum tenens physicians are considered independent contractors. As such, they will receive a 1099 at the end of the year for income reporting, and they will be subject to the federal self-employment tax. In order to avoid paying tax penalties, quarterly tax estimates should be paid. To optimize tax-advantaged savings, many physicians working as independent contractors elect to be taxed as a sole proprietorship or a corporation and open a retirement account such as a solo 401k. One can consult a tax professional or accountant for further advice on this or educate herself via investment resources such as the White Coat Investor (www.whitecoatinvestor.com).

Malpractice coverage is provided through the locum tenens agency, but it is wise to verify that it has standard terms ($1 million/$3 million limits) and to obtain a copy of the certificate of coverage for your own records. Health, dental, and vision benefits are typically not offered to nonemployees (ie, independent contractors), so the locums physician will be responsible for furnishing this on her own.

Practical and Lifestyle Considerations

Traveling across the country (or even the world) to move from one locums assignment to the next may be appealing to the itinerant spirit and appalling to the homebody or introvert. For some otolaryngologists with school-aged children, a family member with special needs, or even a pet to care for, locums work may not be a viable option. Some people are lucky enough to have a spouse and/or children who will come along for the experience, perhaps testing out a new town that they may decide to call home if a permanent position is a possibility. When deciding whether or not to take an assignment, some questions to ask oneself include the following:

- Would I be comfortable getting around this new hospital/town?
- Am I familiar with the EHR system?
- If I have downtime, is there enough around to keep me entertained?
- Will I need childcare while working? If so, what is the availability like in the area?
- With whom will I be working? Will someone be available if I have a question regarding patient care, clinic supplies, hospital logistics, etc.?
- What types of patients will I be seeing? What types of procedures/surgeries will I be expected to perform?

The best way to gain answers to these questions is by speaking with the locums agency recruiter, the clinic manager (if applicable), any staff otolaryngologists currently employed by the hospital/practice, and, if possible, any other physicians who have recently completed a locum tenens assignment there.

Testimonial

After graduating residency in 2017, I moved to Japan to join my husband, a military physician, who had already been overseas for the previous 6 months. We had one son at the time, then 3 years old. After briefly looking into volunteer opportunities at the military hospital and realizing they were quite sparse, I decided to look into locum tenens work. My goals were 3-fold: to earn some income, to maintain my recently acquired skill set, and to figure out what type of position would be a good fit for me long-term.

I was interviewed for 3 positions—one in Alaska, one in West Virginia, and one in Minnesota. In the end, the position in Alaska wanted too much of a recurring commitment for my availability, the West Virginia hospital decided they could not afford a locums physician, and the Minnesota position seemed as a good fit. The hospital was hiring a short-term otolaryngologist to fill in for 1 of their 2 otolaryngologists, who was out on medical leave. I agreed to commit to 2 months, a time period during which my husband would be deployed, and I was able to negotiate a slightly higher rate to help cover childcare costs. I was able to arrange an apartment rather than a hotel room, and I negotiated a 4-wheel drive rental vehicle for the Minnesotan winter roads.

On arriving at the hospital, I was provided with 2 full days of orientation and EHR training. I worked in the operating room for a day with the staff otolaryngologist to serve as a form of proctoring. Then, I got to work and enjoyed a busy, productive 2 months of locums work. When they needed help again the following summer, I happily agreed to come back for a second assignment. I got great exposure to what a hospital-employed practice looks like, met many wonderful people, and kept my surgical skills and clinical acumen sharp.

Conclusion

When choosing a career path in otolaryngology, one might consider locum tenens as an opportunity to sample a practice or locale before deciding where to settle down. It may also be an excellent way to garner some new perspective and experience while between jobs or while unable to commit to a long-term position. Before deciding to pursue locum tenens otolaryngology, it is important to consider logistical and lifestyle factors. When deciding on an assignment, one must consider the proposed work schedule, call obligation, patient acuity, and reimbursement. For some otolaryngologists, serving as a "place holder" can be a rewarding, fun experience that neatly fills a gap in her career path or satisfies a desire to travel, and locum tenens work should not be overlooked or written off by the discerning otolaryngologist.

FINDING THE RIGHT JOB IN OTOLARYNGOLOGY: PRIVATE PRACTICE
Introduction

Private Practice Otolaryngology continues to be a viable option for those completing residency or for seasoned practitioners looking to make a change from military or academic practice. Modern private practice Otolaryngology offers a variety of settings from solo to group practice, or multispecialty group practice, employed private practice, and even locum tenens. Subspecialty trained Otolaryngologists can also find a niche in private practice in 2022. Demographic trends are affecting private practice Otolaryngology. And although these trends are affecting the outward appearance of the private practice model, it is still possible to have a professionally satisfying career in Otolaryngology as a private practitioner. Once the decision for private practice has been made, the challenge will be locating the opportunity that best accommodates all needs for the Otolaryngologist and family. Despite the major landscape shift in private practice Otolaryngology, many positions are available to provide a rewarding career, wellness, intellectual stimulation, collaboration, financial security, and even academic accolades.

Searching for opportunities, interviewing, and contract negotiations are certainly vital ingredients in the private practice recipe. Equally important is knowledge of the forces acting on Otolaryngology at present that create opportunities for private practice employment. Although our specialty is currently driven by outcomes research and published data, it is also true that in this evidence-based era of Otolaryngology, the medical literature is lacking in guidance for locating and securing a private practice position; in fact, the good old fashioned ways of networking, cold-calling, and back-channel communication are still the best ways to find the right opportunity.

Trends in the Otolaryngology Workforce

One of the great benefits of modern Otolaryngology training is the variety of career choices available to those who complete the rigorous process. Following the required years of education, the Otolaryngologist may pick from academic, private, or military positions or may choose to pursue fellowship training in subspecialty areas including Head and Neck Surgery and Reconstruction, Laryngology, Pediatric Otolaryngology, Facial Plastics and Reconstruction, Otology and Neurotology, Rhinology and Skull Base Surgery, and Sleep Surgery.[9] Reasons cited for the pursuit of advanced training include desire for additional expertise in a focused area of Otolaryngology and intellectual challenge of subspecialty practice. However, it is worth considering a major demographic trend occurring in the United States over the last several years that is expected to continue for the foreseeable future: the aging of the population.[10] Aging population affects the Otolaryngology work force in 2 important ways. First, the number of patients needing care is increasing, and second, the number of Otolaryngologists reaching the age of retirement is increasing. The final result is a shortage of Otolaryngologists to provide the care these patients will eventually require. When the shrinking supply of private practice Otolaryngologists is coupled with the increasing trend toward advanced training,[9,10] the end result is an increased opportunity to pursue private practice employment. Private practice is an important variable in the equation of providing care to the aging population, and Comprehensive Otolaryngologists as well as Fellowship Trained Subspecialists can find a home in the private world. Private practice, especially in rural areas, is in short supply, and there is often a need for subspecialty care (most often otology and rhinology) outside of large urban regions.[9]

Another trend shaping the private practice landscape is consolidation.[11] Since the early 2000s, private practice has seen a growing number of smaller practices acquired by larger groups. Large groups can either be single specialty Otolaryngology or multispecialty practices. Large group employment can be classified broadly into the following categories: privately owned, hospital employed and owned, or venture capital owned. Investigate the details of each of these models before you interview or sign a contract, as the function and governance in each of these models is quite different. The once prevalent single Otolaryngologist practice is now a rarity in the United States, and with its disappearance, growth of larger groups concentrated in major metropolitan areas has become more common. Smaller private practices generally offer greater autonomy with more of the administrative burden being borne by the Otolaryngologist who owns the practice.[12] In contrast larger groups generally offer less administrative burden, greater contractual power with insurers, and less on call responsibilities. In the middle are small group Otolaryngology practices typically composed of 2 to 10 Otolaryngologists. Small groups share some of the advantages of both single Otolaryngologist practices and large groups with greater autonomy and less on-call burden but may face challenges with insurance contracts. Either way, you can find the right fit for your practice style and management needs in the private realm in 2021.

There is important discussion throughout our specialty on the topic of diversity. Our leadership is to be commended for facing this important topic with a plan to find a place for everyone in our specialty. Private practitioners have joined our academic colleagues in forming a plan for increasing the ranks of minority physicians in Otolaryngology, serving diverse communities, and building the base of applicants and leaders in Otolaryngology.[13] Private Practitioners have contributed to this effort (several were investigators on the article cited in this paragraph, and one is the AAO-HNSF Immediate Past President), and all Otolaryngologists should be reassured that there is a home in private practice. Dr Denneny and the staff of the American Academy of Otolaryngology-Head and Neck Surgery Foundation (AAO-HNSF) have done a great job of making private practice Otolaryngologists feel welcome at the table of academy leadership.

The myriad effects of the COVID19 pandemic have been well documented throughout the Otolaryngology literature.[14] And although some private practices will endure irreparable harm, others will emerge stronger than ever and will be looking for qualified Otolaryngologists to fill their ranks and provide needed care in their respective communities. Otolaryngologists should see this as an opportunity to find a practice that needs their skills. Private practice has endured many trials, and the pandemic will provide yet another instance for the best private practices to remain at a competitive advantage for hiring the best Otolaryngology applicants.

Identifying Potential Jobs

In "normal" times, most would start a search for private practice jobs at the annual AAO-HNSF Meeting. The Expo Hall typically has a bulletin board dedicated entirely to job postings, including private practice. There would typically be numerous opportunities to discuss these positions with the Otolaryngologists offering them, perhaps even having that first interview. If an in-person gathering cannot take place this fall, then the AAO-HNSF showed their flexibility in 2020 by putting on an excellent virtual meeting with an online Expo Hall and job postings. I would also recommend searching for job postings on the AAO-HNSF Website. As of the date of this writing (May 10, 2021), there were 253 listings for an Otolaryngologist. Not all of these are private practice jobs, but as you search through the listings you will be able to identify private practice opportunities. And keep in mind that as many academic medical centers grow in size and spread out into the community, they become interested in hiring private practice Otolaryngologists to fill those community slots; you could potentially find a position that has academic ties yet be in private practice.

If your online search does not yield results, then schedule an appointment with your program's Chair or Residency Director. These 2 individuals will know where former residents are in practice and whether they are hiring. In our group, we have found that hiring residents who trained at the same program creates a smooth transition into practice and offers new hires something significant in common with other members of the group. This common bond creates collegiality from the start of the professional relationship and helps improve retention.

If you have come to a dead end after online search and discussing potential opportunities with key faculty members at your training facility, then consider cold calling some practices in an area of the country that you would like to live. You can search out the practices in the city of your choice via a search engine or on the AAO-HNSF Website. "Cold calls, word of mouth, and networking with contacts"[15] are still good strategies for finding the right position even in the digital age.

A word of caution with regard to recruiting firms is appropriate here. Although a recruiting firm can make your search for jobs easier, keep in mind that the recruiting firm has its own interests in mind ONLY and not yours: the firm is paid based on placement, not on retention, and thus their sole motivation is securing the commission they receive for having an applicant sign the contract for the job they have located. You could wind up with a fantastic opportunity from a recruiting firm, but you could just as well find yourself relocating if you are not careful in making certain the opportunity is right for you and your family. Beware of the pressure a recruiter will apply to you to take the position they are offering soon after you have interviewed.

The Interview

Once you have located some opportunities you are ready to begin the interview process. An important point on this topic is relevant to consider: the opportunity has to be right for EVERYONE in the equation, the spouse or significant other, the family, and the Otolaryngologist. I located a great opportunity for me with all the things I was looking for in a private practice job, but it was 5 hours from our nearest family members, my wife did not know anyone in the community, nor were there good schools for my kids. This would have been the exact wrong job for us because it did not meet the needs of my spouse nor family.

Different practices will handle the interview process in different ways. If possible, consider a 3-interview technique to make sure the position is the right one for you and your family. The first interview is a get to know one another process where the candidate has a chance to learn about the practice, its culture, and the way the candidate might fit into the current structure and the practice has a chance to find out more about the candidate beyond the resume and references. Make sure during this first interview that the position fits your professional needs: if you desire a practice with a heavy allergy component, verify the Otolaryngologists in the group practice allergy and belong to the American Academy of Otolaryngic Allergy for example. The second interview is for getting into the nuts and bolts of the practice; this is the time to review the practice's finances, their long-term financial stability, identify any potential salary guarantees, and discuss relocation expenses, malpractice premiums, and any other pertinent financial issues—retirement savings, benefits packages, and so forth. Be wary of any practice that is not forthright about their finances and financial position, as this is a major red flag. If the practice is truly interested in you and able to offer you job security, then they should be willing to share financial data with you. The third and final interview is for finishing up any final details and for the candidate to sign the contract of employment. Keep in mind that you are an Otolaryngologist and not a health care nor labor attorney; secure counsel before you sign any agreement to make sure that you and the potential employer are protected in the contract.[15] Your attorney can also counsel you as to whether you need to consult a tax professional or financial planner to assist you in your new employment and relocation.

In an article published in 2014, Richard Quinn lists the 4 Rs of interviewing successfully for medical positions[15]; these are Research, References, Resume, and Roundtable. Research the opportunity; what are the strengths and weaknesses of the practice, what is its reputation in the community, why do they need to add another Otolaryngologist at this time, and what has been their track record of hiring and retaining previous Otolaryngology employees are important topics to investigate. Next, make sure your References are the best ones you can obtain, as your potential employer will be certain to query your references about your character, work ethic, and skills. It is likewise your prerogative to do the same assessment of the employer; a good way is to contact some of the medical colleagues in their community. Having your Resume in order is always important during a job search; if your residency program does not offer resume assistance, then hire a professional to help make your resume true and impressive. Finally, hold a Roundtable with all of the key people involved in your decision; remember to include your family in the decision process and make sure the opportunity is as good for them as it may be for you.

Conclusion

Private practice continues to offer Otolaryngologists an intellectually stimulating, professionally satisfying, and financially secure opportunity. Private practitioners are a vital component of the workforce needed in the United States currently to provide comprehensive care to the aging population. Although the outward appearance of private practice has changed in many ways over the years, private practice continues to be a place where Otolaryngologists can thrive.

DISCLOSURE

The author has nothing to disclose.

CONFLICTS OF INTEREST

AAO-HNSF Rhinology & Allergy Education Committee, AAO-HSNF Legislative Affairs Committee, Stryker ENT Consultant; none of these is a conflict of interest for the production of this article.

REFERENCES

1. Setzen G. Private practice otolaryngology is not a dying concept. Entnet.org Bulletin; 2018. p. 9.
2. Maniscalco MM. A physician's guide to working as a locum tenens. J Am Board Fam Pract 2003;16(3):242–5.
3. Kealey K. 40 years of locum tenens: the origins of a new approach to healthcare. Available at: https://comphealth.com/resources/the-origin-of-locum-tenens/. Accessed May 8, 2021.
4. NALTO: best practice guidelines. Available at: https://www.nalto.org/about. Accessed May 13, 2021.
5. Blumenthal DM, Olenski AR, Tsugawa Y, et al. Association between treatment by locum tenens internal medicine physicians and 30-day mortality among hospitalized medicare beneficiaries. JAMA 2017;318(21):2119–29.

6. Chiu RG, Nunna RS, Siddiqui N, et al. Locum tenens neurosurgery in the United States: a medicare claims analysis of outcomes, complications, and cost of care. World Neurosurg 2020;142:e210–4.

7. Nolan TL, Kandel JJ, Nakayama DK. Quality and extent of locum tenens coverage in pediatric surgical practices. Am Surg 2015;81(4):377–80.

8. Dzhashi V. Finding best locum tenens companies: what I've learned after 5+ years of full-time locums work. Available at: https://thelocumguy.com/best-locum-tenens-companies/. Accessed May 13, 2021.

9. Miller RH, McCrary HC, Gurgel RK. Assessing trends in fellowship training among otolaryngology residents: a national survey study. Otolaryngol Head Neck Surg 2021. https://doi.org/10.1177/0194599821994477.

10. Cass LM, Smith JB. The current state of the otolaryngology workforce. Otolaryngol Clin N Am October 2020;53(5):915–26.

11. Hanson PS. Private practice trends in the us: will increasing competitiveness weaken the profession? Health Management 2009;9(1):1–3.

12. Rapoport SK. This Doctor's appreciation for medicine grew after a move to a small town. Here's how. ENTtoday 2021;16(1):10–2.

13. Truesdale CM, et al. Prioritizing diversity in otolaryngology-head and neck surgery: starting a conversation. Otolaryngol Head Neck Surg 2021;164(2):229–33.

14. Rubin R. COVID-19's crushing effects on medical practices, some of which might not survive. JAMA 2020;324(4):321–3.

15. Quinn R. Landing your first otolaryngology job. ENTtoday 2014;9(9):1–3.

Making a Major Change
Changing Your Practice Setting, Retirement, and Locums

Hosai Todd Hesham, MD[a,b],*, Kenneth Grundfast, MD[c,1],
Kathleen Sarber, MD[d,e]

KEYWORDS

- Career change • Burn-out • Retirement • Locum tenens • Academic medicine
- Private practice

KEY POINTS

- Preparation for both young and experienced physicians would benefit from the preparation and anticipation of career change and career goals.
- Career change may occur due to changes in personal and professional situations and goals.
- Career options, from the government to private practice, to locum tenens are discussed.

INTRODUCTION

"What is your greatest strength?" That is a question that we have answered multiple times in our careers. It is a question that we ask of those who come after us. The answers are often the same. A scripted and choreographed dance to prove that we have the kind of strength that is required for this job, the medical profession, and the profession that at times is our main identity. Although we all know that there is no one best answer, we all answer with confidence. Cardiothoracic surgeon turned palliative care physician during his midcareer, Dr Christopher Strzalka, writes that adaptability is his greatest strength. In fact, he calls adaptability a surgeon's best friend. "The adaptability that is so crucial for patients and their families to adjust to progressive and

[a] Adjunct Faculty, Department of Surgery, Division of Otolaryngology, George Washington University, Washington, DC, USA; [b] Maryland ENT Associates, Privia, Private Practice, Silver Spring, MD, USA; [c] Department of Otolaryngology, Boston University, Boston, MA, USA; [d] Department of Surgery, F. Edward Hebert School of Medicine, Uniformed Services University of the Health Sciences, Bethesda, MD 20814, USA; [e] Department of Otolaryngology–Head and Neck Surgery, Brooke Army Medical Center, 3551 Roger Brooke Drive, Fort Sam Houston, TX 78234, USA
[1] Present address: 830 Harrison Avenue, Suite 1400, Boston, MA 02118.
* Corresponding author. 2415 Musgrove Road, Suite 203, Silver Spring, MD 20904
E-mail address: HosaiHesham@gmail.com

Otolaryngol Clin N Am 55 (2022) 33–41
https://doi.org/10.1016/j.otc.2021.08.010
0030-6665/22/© 2021 Elsevier Inc. All rights reserved.

critical illness is the same quality we need as practitioners to accommodate them." As it turns out, Dr Strzalka is correct in whereby he ranks adaptability when it comes to changes in one's career and transition.[1] Surgeons are often stereotyped as rigid individuals who value consistency and routine. After all, these values are necessary to be a technically good surgeon. Is it the training that molds the surgeon or do these personality types gravitate toward surgery? Regardless of the answer to that question, what we do know is that the same characteristics that make us good surgeons do not necessarily prepare us well for adapting to change.

Change can be painful to a surgeon. We publish on reluctance to change from anecdotal practice to evidence-based practice. We see it in trying to adapt to a new organizational structure or electronic medical records (EMR). Career change is something that most of us rarely think about. One might conclude that the reason many of us continues to work in environments whereby we are not fulfilled or happy is that change is even harder to accept or endure. In addition, we have invested and sacrificed so much just to be in our current position. We learn how to operate, how to take care of patients, and how to interact with our colleagues throughout our training and career. However, we are not well prepared or informed on how to navigate from one practice setting to another. When we do go through a career change, most of these changes occur because it has been forced on us: the hospital is bought by a new entity, your significant other gets a job across the country, a colleague or you get sick, or the most recent example, the COVID-19 pandemic upends clinical practice as we knew it. It is no wonder that many would consider career change an unpleasant topic. Ebberweinn and colleagues noted that study participants who anticipated career change methodically and realistically, even when their jobs seemed to be secure, cited better experiences of the transition and perceived themselves to be coping better than did participants who ignored signs of change or reacted unrealistically soon after the job loss.[2] With this in mind, it would be wise to seek guidance from peers and colleagues regarding our options when it comes to transitions or changes in our career. Perhaps such guidance can result in happier and more fulfilled physicians who continue to feel that they are impactful.

In this article, our aim is to focus on how to prepare for the possibility of needing to make a career transition. We will discuss things to consider when making a transition from unproductive or unfulfilling work or career tract to a position that is more aligned with your values and goals. We propose methodically thinking about these issues as it relates to a career timeline: early career, midcareer, late career, and preparation for retirement. We will focus on the why, how, and potential implications in each phase.

EARLY CAREER

Early in our careers, we tend to go into the type of setting that we thought we would be best suited for based on our training and guidance from mentors. Many times, the ideal practice is not clear and one may settle into a role by default such as continuing at the institution we trained at or going into an employed position or private practice. Most physicians spend only a few years at their first job out of training. A CompHealth 2018 survey found that, although new physicians are largely satisfied in their first positions, few planned to stay long term. Only 37% planned to stay in their first position beyond the end of their contract, 26% planned to move on to something new, and 37% were still undecided about what they want to do.[3] In the same survey, young physicians said compensation (59%), work/life balance (51%), and bad management (45%) were the main reasons they sought new job opportunities. Reasons were significantly different between gender, with men most commonly identifying compensation (69%), whereas women identified poor work/life balance (56%).

Luckily, the transition can be easiest at this phase of one's career for obvious reasons. Despite this fact, many continue working in less-than-ideal circumstances for a variety of reasons ranging from financial concerns, perceived lack of options, or loyalty to their institution or a mentor. In addition, the institutions or practices that hire these young surgeons invest significant resources for onboarding. Considering the facts mentioned thus far, it is critical to mentor otolaryngologists in training about their options early in their professional career. This may lead to informed decision-making that will be beneficial both for the new otolaryngologist and their employer.

Most otolaryngologists who choose to pursue a fellowship do so following residency. Although this may delay building wealth, fellowship salary is usually significantly higher than a resident's earnings. This increase may therefore make the decision to stay in training for 1 or 2 more years easier to accept, especially for those with young families. Once a full clinical salary is earned, however, the transition back to a fellow's salary is much more difficult. A recent survey showed that most otolaryngologists choose to do a fellowship to gain additional expertise beyond residency training (35%) and for the intellectual appeal (30%).[4] Another study showed that those interested in an academic career who were young (<29 years) and with less educational debt tended to be more interested in fellowship.[5] Interestingly, the delay in financial compensation may not be recuperated by most subspecialties. Despite the logical human capital theory, a 2016 report calculated the value of a 30-year career for a general otolaryngologist and 10 subspecialties.[6] This calculation was based on the 2011 data collected in the Socioeconomic Survey Among Members. Only skull base surgery and rhinology held more value in their calculations over a general otolaryngologist, whereas every other recognized subspecialty netted hundreds of thousands of dollars less. The lowest paid subspecialty ("otolaryngologic allergy") netted $3.6 million dollars. This is evidence that all otolaryngologists are well compensated, but if financial gain is a top driver in choosing a career path, then a fellowship should not be a consideration.

For those graduating otolaryngologists who may want more time and opportunity to experience a practice setting before committing, locum tenens may prove worthwhile. Private practices of all sizes as well as the Veterans Affairs system seek occasional, short-term, and longer-term contracts while actively seeking permanent staff to fill the needs of the clinic. Although the hospital has requirements that must be met, clinic and surgery schedules can be negotiated to optimize flexibility. Locums are generally conducted through a contracting agency, although opportunities exist to make an agreement directly with practice. The agency covers malpractice insurance and travel costs, and will assist with credentialing, obtaining state medical license, Drug Enforcement Agency license, and other necessary training as required by the practice. Pay is negotiated by the hour or day for each job taken. Because licenses can be an expensive upfront cost coming out of residency, it could be beneficial to do even a short duration of locums in the state or states that one has decided they will settle in. Downsides to locums work include the need to obtain health care coverage and the lack of employer contribution to retirement pay. Because the physician is considered a contractor and not an employee, taxes become slightly more complicated, but all expenses related to work can be deducted. Traveling to different, often rural, parts of the country may be beneficial for those who have not chosen a geographic location to settle. Conversely, this can be a downside for those whose families must remain at home.

Vickery and colleagues published in 2016 that the average age of male otolaryngologist is 54 and 49 for female otolaryngologists.[7] An aging workforce places a young otolaryngologist in a favorable position. **Fig. 1** Early-career otolaryngologists can use multiple resources to prepare for possible career changes and know when it is time to pursue a change:

1. Use mentors within and outside otolaryngology. The same concept applies to gathering information from academic physicians and physicians in private practice.
2. Stay connected with other colleagues. Be open to discussing compensation, contract negotiation, and sharing resources.
3. Consider additional training or fellowship.
4. Consider locum tenens before committing to a geographic location or institution.
5. Review contracts with colleagues and mentors in addition to an attorney.
6. Create a realistic timeline of career growth. For example, plan to achieve an associate professorship in 5 years or have a contractually agreed-on transition when a senior partner retires.
7. Take advantage of business management and coding seminars and courses.
8. Continue to network. Join the local medical society and otolaryngology groups.

MIDCAREER

There are many reasons for a professional transition during midcareer phase. Many choose to make a transition to pursue academic or leadership advancement. Others may want to focus on a practice niche and find that changing geographic location or organization type may be necessary to achieve this. Finally, a significant number of midcareer clinicians change due to burnout, feeling unappreciated, financial dissatisfaction, divorce, or family issues.

Bickel and colleagues provide techniques that academic health systems (AHSs) can adopt to assist midcareer clinicians in growth. "Continuing engagement of midcareer faculty is critical to the functioning of AHSs." However, despite their strong desire for ongoing meaningful work, many midcareer faculties are at a standstill, with further promotion unlikely. Drawing on more than 40 years of working closely with AHS faculty, the author describes growth-promoting strategies that midcareer faculty can tailor to individual needs, including questions for personal reflection. Research on adult development and resilience indicates that reexamining commitments at this career stage is healthy and begins with individuals taking a fresh look at what they value

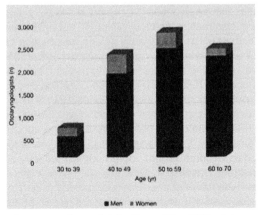

Fig. 1. Graph shows the age and sex distribution of the 8104 otolaryngologists for whom data on both age and sex were available.

most. When individuals shift attention from constraints to those aspects of themselves and their situations that they can modify, they often discern new possibilities and become more agile. AHSs also can do a great deal to assist faculty with adjustments inherent in this midlife stage.[8]

Unfortunately, many midcareer otolaryngologists feel unsupported and find themselves in situations whereby they feel a transition may be necessary. Many choose to find academic institutions whereby they feel valued based on what they can bring to the program. Others may decide to leave academic medicine to an employed hospital or private practice position.

In relation to academic practice, the midcareer is a common and practical phase whereby many women otolaryngologists return to academic medicine. Tradition has held that academic productivity among women physicians exponentially increases during their midcareer phase. However, a recent study showed that early-career female otolaryngologists are keeping pace with their male counterparts in publication productivity within some subspecialties.[9] The constraints of work–life balance and family planning impact academic productivity of early-career women in medicine. However, this loss is recuperated and more during their mid entering to late career.[10–12]

Another practical reason for a career transition is moving to a setting whereby one has more access to a particular patient population. An example would be after several years in general practice, one might find a particular desire to focus exclusively on patients with sinus disease or sleep apnea. A move to a new location or a different practice whereby that expertise is lacking may make that transition easier.

Finally, burnout and dissatisfaction may lead to an unplanned career transition during midcareer. A recently published research letter identified an association between burnout and the likelihood of leaving the organization among physicians in a broad spectrum of specialties at the Cleveland Clinic.[13] Within otolaryngology, burnout is more common among academic otolaryngologists than those outside of academic medicine. However, there might be research bias as most of the published research focuses on academia. Women experienced a statistically higher level of emotional exhaustion than men. In addition, associate professors were significantly more burned out than full professors and microvascular surgeons were notably more burned out than all other subspecialists. The strongest predictors of burnout were dissatisfaction with the balance between personal and professional life, low professional self-worth, inadequate research time, and inadequate administration time. A significant association was seen between high burnout and the likelihood to leave academic medicine within the next 1 to 2 years.[14]

Locum tenens work may be a reasonable option to either bridge the financial gap after an unplanned exit from a position or to explore other clinical practices that could be a better fit with one's personal and professional goals. Downsides to locum tenens work in midcareer may be the negative connotation of a locum physician. A survey of health care team members found that locums were often perceived to be inferior to permanent physicians in terms of competency, quality, and safety.[15] This perception is false, however. A United States review of Medicare beneficiaries undergoing neurosurgery found no significant difference in mortality, complication rate, hospital stay, or cost between permanently employed versus locum tenens neurosurgeons.[16] (The author (KS) has not encountered this negative perception in her experience at 4 different practice locations over the last 7 years.) Locum physicians are also considered "outside" of the institution and thus do not participate or have a voice in organizational decisions. Conversely, a break from administrative and hierarchical politics could provide a much-needed respite as well as some perspective on what values and contributions one truly desires in their next career move.

Midcareer can be a time of introspection and formative thinking as physicians contemplate their level of satisfaction with what they are currently doing and give thought to new things they might want to do. Midcareer is a time when physicians often give thought to what they will want to do during the latter part of their career. Some are content to continue doing in the future what they have conducted in the past while looking forward to retirement with time to pursue hobbies and recreational activities. Some begin to think about doing something different. For those who contemplate making a change, some intermittently think of what things might be like if they were to make a change—but they never actually make a change. Others begin to give progressively more thought to the practical aspect of really making a change. Changes can occur in many ways. Some who have spent most of their professional lives in private practice may want to begin participating in teaching, and some who have spent their professional lives in the world of academic medicine may decide that they would prefer to be in private practice. Some physicians who have come to the realization that they have administrative skills may aspire to move into positions in which they can use their administrative skills for a certain portion of their time devoting the remainder of their time to continuing in the practice of medicine.

Although making a change at midcareer can be exciting and enticing, such change can be fraught with challenges. Common challenges include potential financial hardship, the potential need for geographic relocation, and the psychological fear of not succeeding or becoming unhappy after a change is made.

Even though making a change can be daunting, change can be made and can be exciting as well as professionally rewarding. Some advice for those contemplating making a change:

- Introspection to identify the impetus for making a change:

What are the reasons for wanting to make a change? Is the desire to change stemming from dissatisfaction, boredom, or a feeling that you have skills and intellect that you are not currently using but you want to use ? Do you want to enhance your income? Maybe you have reached a plateau in your current situation, and you think you could earn more in a newer situation. Introspection and contemplation can go on for a very long time without any action being taken or can lead to a next step.

- Assessment of skills:

Have you developed special expertise, perhaps a technical, or surgical skill or maybe skills in management or administration? If you have in the past accepted administrative responsibilities, conducted a good job with administrative work, and enjoyed doing it, you might want to move into a position in which you are given significant administrative responsibilities for which you will be paid, such as being a chief medical officer or a quality assurance officer. If you are on the faculty of a medical school, you might aspire to hold the position of assistant dean, or dean at the medical school. Have you realized that you like to teach and work with young people? Perhaps you would like to volunteer to get involved in teaching medical students, residents, and advanced practice providers. Maybe instead of volunteering, you would like to become a full-time member of the faculty at a medical school.

- Exploring possibilities:

The key to actually making a change for the latter portion of a career is networking. By the time you have gotten to midcareer, you know a lot of people with whom you have common interests and who likely will be eager to be of help to you, not only giving you advice but also putting you in touch with those who can offer you positions that enable you to make the change you are seeking. Finding a new opportunity that meets your need for a change can take time, so the sooner you begin networking and the wider your net, the more likely you will be to find the opportunity you are seeking.

- Stepwise approach:

A common impediment to making a change is the incorrect assumption that the change has to be abrupt and climactic. This is not true. Often, the most successful changes made midcareer are the changes that occur incrementally over time. For example, the physician in private practice who desires to spend time teaching can make a transition by volunteering to teach part time, perhaps 1 day each week, then increase time spent teaching and decrease time devoted to patient care over several years. Similarly, the physician who is a full-time faculty member who aspires to hold a dean position can increase time spent on school of medicine activities while decreasing the amount of time spent operating and seeing patients.

LATE CAREER AND PREPARATION FOR RETIREMENT

A 2017 AAO-HNS survey found that that the mean expected retirement age among otolaryngologists is 67.[17] Accurate data, however, are not readily available and it is thought that physicians, in general, retire later than the general population. Dr Robert Sataloff writes the following regarding physicians and retirement:

"Several factors have been identified that influence delay in retirement among physicians. These include flexibility of work hours, intensity of work hours, work satisfaction, other career opportunities (or lack thereof), resource adequacy, sense of intrinsic self-worth, convenience, financial incentives, relationships with coworkers, length of training and late entry into the workforce, attachment to work and related strong work identity, and the 4% rule. The 4% rule says that a person will need approximately 25 times his/her annual expenses in savings/investments to retire with a comfortable lifestyle over a 30-year period (anticipating that investments will yield 4% per year). For many physicians, it is difficult to save enough money to afford to retire comfortably using this equation; and the 4% rule can be affected adversely by substantial market downturns, and by longevity greater than 30 years."[18]

Aside from economic considerations, there are many other topics to consider when planning for retirement during late-career phase. Most late-career otolaryngologists enjoy stability in their practice setting. Whether that stability comes with work satisfaction or not is a different story. Lack of satisfaction may result in early retirement, especially if economic factors are not a concern. In many cases, we encounter private practice or academic otolaryngologists with reasonable work satisfaction and stability without a clear idea of when or how to retire. Gradual planning for retirement should take into account physical ability and impairment, psychosocial adjustment, alternative contributions to the field, and economic factors.

American College of Surgeons issued a statement regarding the "Aging Surgeon" in 2016.[19] The ACS does not favor a mandatory retirement age because the onset and rate of age-related decline in clinical performance vary among individuals. The ACS believes that a mandatory retirement age may have a deleterious impact on access to experienced surgical care, particularly in rural and underserved areas. Objective assessment of fitness should supplant consideration of a mandatory retirement age. Institutions are recommended to develop a process through which surgeons are evaluated starting at age 65 to 70. Surgeons undergo voluntary and confidential baseline physical examination and visual testing by their personal physician for overall health assessment. Regular interval reevaluation thereafter is prudent for those without identifiable issues on the index examination. Surgeons are encouraged to also voluntarily assess their neurocognitive function using confidential online tools. As a part of one's professional obligation, voluntary self-disclosure of any concerning and validated findings is encouraged, and limitations of activities may be appropriate. Otolaryngologists have the benefit of stopping surgical practice and continuing to practice medicine. Older surgeons provide immense teaching and mentoring resources to the otolaryngologic community. In addition, otolaryngologists near retirement or those that have decreased surgical practice can provide much-needed medical care in underserved areas such as Indian Health Services, Veterans Administration, or global health. Finally, contribution to medical education is not limited to otolaryngology only. Many late-career otolaryngologists can contribute to medical school education or advanced practitioner training. Other examples of continued involvement in the medical field are hospital administration positions, consultants for EMR systems, independent medical review, hospital informatics, and many others. These alternative contributions to the medical field may not come with equal monetary contribution; however, these opportunities provide purpose and fulfillment to many. Finally, if the decision to step away from clinical practice was made too early, or if one's retirement location is different than their current practice, locum tenens could provide flexible practice at a pace and time that is, less demanding.

Transition out of clinical and surgical practice does not need to be sudden and full stop. It can be deliberate and gradual. The transition also does not mean a lack of productivity. With thought and planning, this next phase of one's life can be immensely fruitful and satisfying.

SUMMARY

Career transitions can be much more successful if planned deliberately and thoughtfully. Considerations are different among early-career, midcareer, and retirement age otolaryngologists. Using available resources, professional networks, and mentors can be extremely helpful.

DISCLOSURE

The authors have nothing to disclose.

REFERENCES

1. Strzalka, C. Adaptability is the surgeon's best friend. MDedge.com, July 9, 2014.
2. Ebberwein CA, Krieshok TS, Ulven JC, et al. Voices in transition: Lessons on career adaptability. Career Dev Q 2004;52(4):292–308.
3. Survey Report: Millennial doctors still finding jobs the old-fashioned way. CompHealth Blog 2018.
4. Miller RH, McCrary HC, Gurgel RK. Assessing Trends in Fellowship Training Among Otolaryngology Residents: A National Survey Study. Otolaryngol Head Neck Surg 2021. https://doi.org/10.1177/0194599821994477. 0194599821994477.
5. Wilson MN, Vila PM, Cohen DS, et al. The pursuit of otolaryngology subspecialty fellowships. Otolaryngol Head Neck Surg 2016;154(6):1027–33.
6. Hull BP, Darrow DH, Derkay CS. The financial value of fellowship training in otolaryngology. Otolaryngol Head Neck Surg 2013;148(6):906–11.

7. Vickery TW, Weterings R, Cabrera-Muffly C. Geographic distribution of otolaryngologists in the United States. Ear. Nose Throat J 2016;95(6):218–23.
8. Bickel J. Not too late to reinvigorate: How midcareer faculty can continue growing. Acad Med 2016;91(12):1601–5.
9. Okafor S, Tibbetts K, Shah G, et al. Is the gender gap closing in otolaryngology subspecialties? An analysis of research productivity. Laryngoscope 2020;130(5): 1144–50.
10. Eloy JA, Svider P, Chandrasekhar SS, et al. Gender disparities in scholarly productivity within academic otolaryngology departments. Otolaryngol Head Neck Surg 2013;148(2):215–22.
11. Eloy JA, Svider PF, Cherla DV, et al. Gender disparities in research productivity among 9952 academic physicians. Laryngoscope 2013;123(8):1865–75.
12. Reed DA, Enders F, Lindor R, et al. Gender differences in academic productivity and leadership appointments of physicians throughout academic careers. Acad Med 2011;86(1):43–7.
13. Windover AK, Martinez K, Mercer MB, et al. Correlates and outcomes of physician burnout within a large academic medical center. JAMA Intern Med 2018; 178(6):856–8.
14. Golub JS, Johns MM III, Weiss PS, et al. Burnout in academic faculty of otolaryngology—Head and neck surgery. Laryngoscope 2008;118(11):1951–6.
15. Ferguson J, Tazzyman A, Walshe K, et al. 'You're just a locum': professional identity and temporary workers in the medical profession. Sociol Health Illness 2021; 43(1):149–66.
16. Chiu RG, Khalid SI, Nunna RS, et al. Locum Tenens Neurosurgery in the United States: A Nationwide Analysis of Outcomes, Complications and Cost of Care. Neurosurgery 2020;67(Supplement_1). nyaa447_166.
17. 2017 AAOHNS Socioeconomic Survey and AOA Practice Benchmarking survey. Available at: https://www.entnet.org/wp-content/uploads/2021/04/2017_SocioeconomicSurvey_v5.pdf.
18. Sataloff RT. Physicians and Retirement. Ear. Nose Throat J 2019;98(7):394–5.
19. Statement on Aging Surgeon. ACS. 2016. Available at: https://www.facs.org/about-acs/statements/80-aging-surgeon.

Honesty and Transparency, Indispensable to the Clinical Mission—Part I

How Tiered Professionalism Interventions Support Teamwork and Prevent Adverse Events

Michael J. Brenner, MD[a,b,*], Richard C. Boothman, JD[c,d,e],
Cynda Hylton Rushton, PhD, MSN, RN[f,g,h],
Carol R. Bradford, MD, MS[i,j], Gerald B. Hickson, MD[e,k]

KEYWORDS

- Professionalism • Teamwork • Surgery • Malpractice risk • Patient safety
- Quality improvement • High reliability • Business of medicine

KEY POINTS

- Many medical and surgical errors cast as "unavoidable" may be preventable by a central, overriding sense of urgency around patient safety, clinical excellence, and high reliability.
- High reliability—the ability to operate in complex, high-hazard domains for extended periods without serious accidents—requires prioritizing safety over other performance pressures.
- The surgeon-as-captain-of-the-ship concept is an anachronistic relic that is antithetical to high reliability and should be supplanted by a commitment to healthcare-as-a-team-sport.
- Tiered professionalism interventions promote teamwork, improve safety, and reduce litigation risk by systematically identifying, measuring, and addressing unprofessional behaviors.
- Achieving high reliability requires honesty—the starting point to just culture, teamwork, and learning systems for investigating and responding to the system side and human side of errors.

[a] Department of Otolaryngology-Head & Neck Surgery, University of Michigan School of Medicine, 1500 East Medical Center Drive SPC 5312, 1904 Taubman Center, Ann Arbor, MI 48109-5312, USA; [b] GTC Quality Improvement Collaborative, Durham, NC, USA; [c] Boothman Consulting Group, LLC, Ann Arbor, MI, USA; [d] Department of Surgery, University of Michigan Medical School, Ann Arbor; [e] Center for Patient and Professional Advocacy, Vanderbilt University Medical Center, Nashville, TN, USA; [f] Johns Hopkins University School of Nursing, Baltimore, MD, USA; [g] Department of Pediatrics, Johns Hopkins University School of Medicine, Baltimore, MD, USA; [h] Berman Institute of Bioethics, Johns Hopkins University School of Medicine, Baltimore, MD, USA; [i] The College of Medicine and James Cancer Hospital and Solove Research Institute; [j] Department of Otolaryngology–Head and Neck Surgery, The Ohio State University Wexner Medical Center, Columbus; [k] Center for Quality, Safety and Risk Prevention, Vanderbilt University Medical Center, Nashville, TN, USA
* Corresponding author.
E-mail address: mbren@med.umich.edu

Otolaryngol Clin N Am 55 (2022) 43–61
https://doi.org/10.1016/j.otc.2021.07.016
0030-6665/22/© 2021 Elsevier Inc. All rights reserved.

Honesty and transparency make you vulnerable. Be honest and transparent anyway.

—Saint Teresa of Calcutta (Mother Teresa)

INTRODUCTION

The *Business of Medicine* includes delivery of safe, effective, and compassionate care with honesty and integrity. Health care organizations that prioritize economics (which are inherently transactional) before core values (which are inherently foundational), often lose focus and invite inconsistency of purpose. The most important competitive business advantage is consistent high quality—achieve that and other factors like financial integrity tend to follow.[1] Relative to other enterprises, core values are particularly important in the profession of health care—whose practitioners are often drawn to the field out of a sense of calling or desire to serve; where the stakes are higher than other fields; and where the success of interventions and the prevention of harm—physical and psychological—rely on carefully orchestrated teams.

Clinical excellence across the continuum of care requires a steadfast commitment to *patient centricity*, defined as "Putting the patient first in an open and sustained engagement of the patient to respectfully and compassionately achieve the best experience and outcome for that person and their family."[2] This aspirational goal emphasizes respectful, accountable, and professional care, and success is predicated on honesty and openness with patients and families. There is also growing awareness of our shared humanity and that the social contract is not unidirectional; relational integrity necessitates attention to the well-being of health professionals and care partners, as articulated in the Declaration for Human Experience.[3] Nowhere is our character more tested than in moments of crisis[4] and when a patient suffers unintended harm.[5,6]

Interspersed through this 3-part series is a vignette that illustrates key points about how harm may arise; how to do right by those who have suffered; and how to prevent future harm—both for the health care team and for the next patient who walks in the door. Professionalism is an essential safeguard to the clinical trapeze that swings over the imperfect netting of clinical care delivery systems. Attention to 3 areas can advance the clinical mission: (1) an expectation of professionalism, (2) a commitment to honesty and transparency throughout the continuum of the patient-professional relationship, and (3) attention to the wellness and resilience of the health care team (**Fig. 1**). In this article, Part 1, we examine the first of these pillars of advancing the clinical mission: *promoting professionalism and teamwork*.

Consider the Following Hypothetical Case

Mr Peyshent is a 68-year-old man having surgery under sedation to reconstruct a nasal defect, which remains after a Mohs micrographic excision of a large cutaneous nasal carcinoma. The patient has obstructive sleep apnea, chronic obstructive pulmonary disease, and is on clopidogrel for cardiac stents. After induction of sedation anesthesia, the attending surgeon, Dr Scalpelle, tries to inject the surgical site with a local anesthetic, but the patient winces and withdraws. Dr Scalpelle glares at the anesthesia resident, Dr Lerner, but says nothing. Dr Lerner anxiously tries to deepen sedation, but the patient begins coughing violently. Dr Scalpelle declares sharply, "I need the patient deeper. Please get your attending!" Visibly rattled, Dr Lerner calls his attending, Dr Propofal. Dr Lerner is leery about deepening sedation too quickly given the patient's sleep apnea, but the last thing he wants is to further upset Dr Scalpelle; so, he pushes a bolus of sedative and increases the oxygen flow. Moments later, the patient becomes apneic, and oxygen saturations plummet. Dr Scalpelle's trainee, Dr Resedent

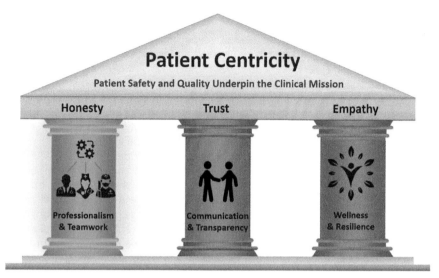

Fig. 1. Values-driven framework for improving honesty and transparency around adverse events. Honesty, trust, and empathy reflect the core values of the health profession promoting safe, high-quality care, and patient centricity. Preventing and responding to patient harm with integrity is supported by 3 pillars.

- *Professionalism and Teamwork (Part 1)* is the focus of the present article. Its touchstones are truth-telling, accountability, and curiosity—pausing to reflect on why unexpected events occur, pinpointing contributing factors, and implementing tiered professionalism interventions tailored to specific needs.
- *Communication and Transparency (Part 2)* offers a principled and comprehensive approach for responding to patient harm. It requires an overriding leadership commitment to honesty and transparency, and it aligns people, organization, and learning systems to achieve just outcomes for patients and families.
- *Wellness and Resilience (Part 3)* is the culmination of the preceding parts. It probes the human dimension of working at the sharp end of care, exploring our shared humanity and relational integrity. After defining the drivers of burnout and moral injury, we describe how leaders can create the path to wellness and resilience.

snaps at Nurse Corage, anxious to gain better access to the patient's airway. The nurse recoils. Dr Resedent performs a jaw thrust to restore breathing and oxygenation.

Reflect on a Few Questions

- How can abrasive interactions undermine patient safety in the operating room?
- Could incivility or unprofessional behavior affect a learner's performance?
- What unspoken lessons are the 2 residents likely to take away from these experiences?
- Whose responsibility is it to identify and address unacceptable behaviors in health care?

The following discussion will examine these questions, explore the link between professionalism and safety, and introduce strategies for supporting professional accountability.

WHAT DEFINES AN ACCOUNTABLE PROFESSIONAL?

Accountability is a willingness to accept responsibility for one's actions, and an accountable professional is one who embodies professionalism—possessing a clear focus on the patient's well-being and that of coworkers, a clear recognition of the importance of culture, and a commitment to technical excellence and staying current in one's specialty. Kirch describes that professionalism engenders, "a culture that is grounded in the values of collaboration, trust and shared accountability.... that encourages transparency and inclusivity, rather than exclusivity.... that is driven equally by our traditional commitment to excellence, and by service to others."[7]

Respect is woven through professionalism—not just for patients and fellow team members but also respect for established practices that improve safety, such as washing our hands, honoring the time out, following established surgical bundles, wearing mask in a pandemic, or getting vaccinated. These seemingly small acts of respect benefit patients and professionals who may otherwise get that infection, which shows up only later after a patient is discharged or a coworker falls ill. Professionalism defines a host of motivational, behavioral, and performance expectations for health care professionals truly committed to patient centricity and clinical excellence. Some of these elements are clinical acumen and technical mastery; pursuit of effective teamwork and communication; and compassion, empathy, and relational integrity for patients, families, and fellow health care team members (**Fig. 2**).

Professionalism is the compass that points true north, allowing us to navigate nuanced ethical dilemmas and moments of crisis. Professionalism is also how we inspire excellence in our learners and confidence in our patients—and it requires intentionality around honesty and transparency. Research finds that when an attending surgeon role models silence, disclosure training has no positive impact on learners' willingness to disclose an error.[8] Professionalism ultimately fosters a culture of patient safety, setting the tone and high baseline expectations for us to embrace surgery-as-a-team rather than surgeon as captain-of-the-ship.

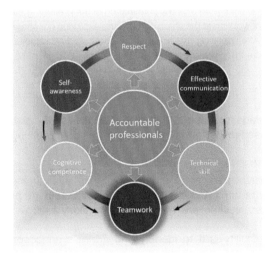

Fig. 2. How accountable professionals promote teamwork. Accountable professionals demonstrate professionalism, which begins with respect for others. The cascading roles of self-awareness, communication, knowledge, and skill allow for effective teamwork and delivery of safe, effective care. *From* Joint Commission Resources.

HOW DO SLIPS OR LAPSES IN PROFESSIONALISM AFFECT PATIENTS AND TEAMS?

After one recognizes the primacy of professionalism, the deleterious and potentially catastrophic effects of unprofessional behavior assume newfound significance. The risk of an emergent airway intervention presented in the case is but one example of how conflict driven by lapses in professionalism can undermine safety. Surgical site infections, stroke, cardiac arrest, and septic shock are all more likely in patients under care of a disruptive clinician.[9,10] Merely witnessing incivility is sufficient to degrade clinical performance and erode trust. Disrespectful behavior is associated with medical error, patient dissatisfaction, and preventable harm. Erosion of team morale also may affect patient and health care professional safety. Team members may experience diminished joy in work, burnout, depression/anxiety, moral distress, and suicidal ideation.[11–13] The latter themes are examined in Part 3 of this trilogy.

Consider again the case of Dr Scalpelle. Did risky acts occur because the microculture was not right in the first place? If the culture had been right, would other team members have been prepared to address the first lapse with a gentle statement ("Dr Scalpelle, let me have a moment to make the patients a bit sleepier," or "Dr Scalpelle, I am concerned…"). These statements are not easily volunteered when they are likely to generate an angry or eye-rolling response. Is it reasonable that Dr Lerner felt compelled to deepen sedation to the point of apnea? When Dr Scalpelle is allowed, day in and day out, to interact in a manner that is dismissive and disrespectful, it dials up the heat on others, who then are prompted to dial up the oxygen—one of the cascading events setting stage for risk of fire today, tomorrow, and the day after that. And it creates a next generation of surgeons who have Dr Scalpelle as a role model.

Medical errors seldom arise from a single point of failure; rather, they usually reflect a complex interplay of how individual medical professionals interact with one another, how they communicate with patients and family members, and how small things can slip through the cracks of imperfect systems. Professionalism affords a baseline of behaviors that create safeguards where imperfect systems cannot always deliver ideal circumstances whenever the unexpected is encountered. Surgeons often expect a team that is well-versed in their specialty and preferences, but what they get often looks closer to pick-up basketball. Amy Edmonson describes "Teamwork on the Fly," observing how diverse specialties increasingly need to come together.[14] In these situations, it becomes even more important to expect professionalism and respect from all members—especially Dr Scalpelle.

Enlightened surgeons recognize that professionalism allows a team to perform safe surgery in less-than-ideal circumstances. A professional graciously accepts the partnership of new, less experienced entrants to the team, showing respect, communicating effectively, and keeping the patient's interest central. Professionalism creates consistency in team performance where it would otherwise not exist. Most surgeons desire a dedicated, highly specialized operating room team—a team that knows the procedure and equipment cold and that can virtually read the surgeon's mind. But this ideal is seldom practical or realistic. Professionalism smooths the jagged edges of erratic care processes, helping to compensate for imperfect systems and to adapt to crises. And safety benefits are not limited to surgery. Professionalism helps navigate complexities of care, ensuring that the patient with cancer does not get "lost in the system."

HOW DO TRAUMATIC LEARNING EXPERIENCES AFFECT PROFESSIONALS?

How faculty and medical leaders interact with learners or new medical group members constitutes an unwritten curriculum whose lessons are taught for a lifetime.[15] When the messaging is to "lay low" and "avoid making waves," open communication and transparency predictably suffer. Conversely, when the culture fosters trust, structural competency, and cultural humility, learning flourishes.[16,17] Traumatic learning experiences—whether stinging criticism, acts of exclusion, or humiliation—may occur in operating rooms, hospital wards, or morbidity and mortality conferences. Unspoken lessons—to be silent, to not admit to being wrong, to honor the hierarchy—leave an indelible mark on the psyches of learners, often reinforced by cultural cues that extol the virtues of silent stoicism.

Danielle Ofri, M.D.'s reflection on her own reluctance to speak out is revealing:

> As a third-year medical student, I once assisted on a late-night operation when suddenly the surgeon's needle accidentally pricked my finger…. I couldn't muster the strength to push back against the hierarchy's deafening silence from my lowly perch as a medical student. That I left my wounded finger submerged in blood for the duration of the surgery during the height of the AIDS epidemic… gives you an inkling of just how hard it is to speak up when the system expects you to shut up and not make trouble.[18]

The lack of psychological safety inculcated during medical school may pervade residency and persist throughout a career. Such was the case for Ofri, who later recounts her reaction to the discovery that she missed the diagnosis of an intracranial bleed on a computed tomography scan. Her reaction was the result of a traumatic learning experience, and though the intracranial bleed was identified by another clinician, it nonetheless took 20 years for her to muster the courage to disclose even a near miss that caused no patient harm. She describes her internal struggle:

> My error – relying on a verbal report rather than looking at the scan itself–was still an error… I was so ashamed that I had given substandard care that I did not tell a soul… I was so devastated that I could hardly function. As a fledgling physician, I felt I had failed my patients so gravely that I was ready to quit medicine altogether. I was not surprised, years later, to read of a nurse who took her own life after an accidental miscalculation of the medication [resulted in death of] an infant in her care.[18]

Such reactions are common in a culture that engenders shame and self-doubt to the detriment of learning and growth. Traumatic learning is experienced by all members of the health care team; nurses, physicians, surgeons, and all allied health professionals are often haunted by the chasm between the care they aspire to provide and the harm that they may cause or witness.

Some readers may not recognize their own experiences—instances where they have been either recipients or the deliverers of the trauma. All professionals should pause on occasion to reflect on performance and to recognize those traumatic disturbances that can keep us, or others who have experienced such disturbances at our hands, from reporting events, speaking up, disclosing errors, and sleeping at night. The *Silence Kills* study, a national survey of more than 1500 interprofessional health care workers, identified several areas that health care professionals find difficult to broach: broken rules, mistakes, lack of support, incompetence, poor teamwork, disrespect, and micromanagement—84% of physicians and 62% of nurses or other clinicians reported seeing coworkers take potentially dangerous shortcuts, but *fewer than 10%* confronted their colleagues with their concerns.[19]

HOW DOES PSYCHOLOGICAL SAFETY RELATE TO TEAM PERFORMANCE?

The importance of psychological safety was powerfully illustrated by *Project Aristotle,* a study by Google that dove deep to understand why some teams were wildly successful, and others languish. The researchers identified 180 teams (115 project teams in engineering and 65 pods in sales) and tested team composition and team dynamics, conducting literally hundreds of double-blinded interviews and aggregating over 250 items from Google's longitudinal study on work and life or engagement surveys. They analyzed the data using 35 statistical models across hundreds of variables to identify what accounts for strong team performance. The most important factor was *psychological safety*, defined as "Team members feel safe to take risks and be vulnerable in front of each other," followed by dependability, role clarity, meaning in the work, and impact (**Fig. 3**).[20] In health care, willingness to take the risk of speaking up is one of the most important ways for teams to improve performance.

A similar conclusion was reached by Lencioni, a renowned expert on organizational health and team management. He is best known as author of *The Five Dysfunctions of a Team,* in which he observes that the most foundational dysfunction is the absence of trust. The bottom of the pyramid of teamwork notes that, "teamwork is founded on vulnerability."[21] Edmondson, a scholar on psychological safety, has been exploring this relationship for more than two decades.[22] Psychological safety needs to be sufficiently embedded in the culture that individuals need not fear retribution if they speak up to raise a concern, ask for help, or identify an opportunity to improve safety. It is imperative that any member of the team can "stop the line." We say that we pursue high reliability and want a learning system; but we cannot get there without making a habit of reporting and recognizing the importance of personal accountability.

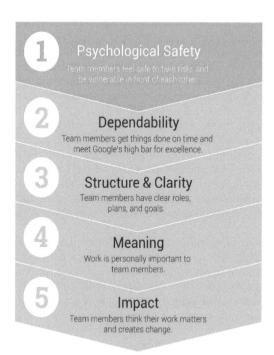

Fig. 3. Psychological safety and team performance. Google's Project Aristotle analyzed 180 teams, finding that psychological safety was the characteristic that most separated high-performing teams from low-performing teams. Reproduced with permission. Credit: Google.

While pressures to stay silent after an error persist, just the opposite is needed to uncover what really happened, to correct faulty systems, to address human error, and to do the right thing for patients and their families at every step along the road. A safety culture can foster joy and meaning in work, as discussed more extensively in Part 3 of this series. When team members have confidence that unprofessional behavior will be consistently addressed in a manner that is purposeful and equitably applied across all health care professionals, the team is motivated to report incidents, and everyone derives greater satisfaction from collaboration. Teamwork is protective against burnout and moral trauma. Failure to adopt these practices places patients at risk for errors, increases turnover, and raises the probability that Dr Scalpelle walks into another room and threatens others.

WHAT IS THE LINK BETWEEN PATIENT COMPLAINTS, SAFETY, AND RISK OF LITIGATION?

In the late 1980s, a research team at Vanderbilt seeking to define the malpractice experience of Florida physicians identified that a small subset of physicians by specialty (2%–8%) accounted for a disproportionate share of claims and payouts. A series of studies followed, seeking to define how these physicians differed from their peers and how to improve their performance. The work identified that high-risk claim experience was not related to the complexity of care delivered but rather to how families assessed their experiences within these high-risk practices. One study taking advantage of unsolicited patient observations/complaints documented by a hospital's office of patient relations found a strong link between unsolicited patient complaints and malpractice litigation.[23]

As this work expanded to collect data across hundreds of institutions, a consistent finding was that an unexpectedly small percentage of clinicians account for a preponderance of complaints by patients. Just 5% of professionals are associated with 35% of unsolicited complaints and 50% of claims dollars; in contrast, almost half of professionals are associated with no unsolicited complaints and 4% of claims dollars. This nonrandom distribution raised the possibility of identifying unprofessional behaviors and intervening to alter these behaviors to improve safety and reduce malpractice claims. This work expanded to coworker observations and demonstrated that patients who receive care from surgeons who model disrespect are more likely to experience avoidable outcomes from surgical site infections, returns to an ICU, reintubation, and a host of medical complications including pneumonia, sepsis, embolism, and stroke.[24,25] Unsolicited patient complaints and coworker observations afford insights across all specialties, including otolaryngology,[26] and representative examples are shown in **Fig. 4**.

Consider again the microculture and interactions depicted in our case. What might have changed if a robust reporting system were in place, if the culture normalized coworkers using the system to reporting concerns, and if the reports were consistently shared? Likely, one of the previous contentious exchanges that Dr Propofal observed between Dr Scalpelle and other team members over years would have drawn attention earlier and prompted timely sharing of concerns. This communication would prompt self-reflection and change; or, if Dr Scalpelle appears unwilling or unable to change, it would prompt an appropriate escalation of response that would be to the benefit of Dr Scalpelle, the team, and the patient. Perhaps the very existence of such infrastructure, with its attendant expectations, would improve behavior. Professionals have a commitment to self-regulate and to collaborate in efforts to group regulate. Failure to do increase the risk of untoward events.

Culture of Reporting Uncovers Latent Safety Threats

Unsolicited Patient Complaints	Co-Worker Observations
"Overheard Dr YY and the Anesthesiologist arguing about why the Dopamine drip had not been hung...the Anesthesiologist stated that it was a waste of medication and "If he (patient) crashes, I'll just do chest compressions."	*"We were going to time out and I turned off the music... Dr XX told me to turn it back on.....I said I can't hear when it is on... He then yelled, please get me a %^&#@ nurse who can hear."*
"There was obviously no communication between my internist and surgeon and absolutely no coordination of care...the physicians keep pointing fingers at each other. I never felt safe."	*"Nurse reported: Dr XX insisted that he would not complete the med rec for discharge..." I'm not 'reinventing the wheel' ... if not discharged it is on YOU!"*
"I don't know what's up with Dr XX... He came busting into the room at 6am and was gone before we could ask him any questions about what is next.... Since my treatment does not seem to be working... I want to know if I am eligible for any trials..."	*"I suggested the family had questions about follow up care, Dr XX stated, "I am not a social worker, it is not my job to talk to the family".* *"I asked Dr XX to pause before closing because we had no tech to do a count with...completely ignored me, grabbed sutures and started to close."*

Fig. 4. Role of patient and coworker reports. Unsolicited patient complaints and coworker observations provide valuable data for identifying and responding to potential areas of concern.

HOW DO TIERED INTERVENTIONS PROMOTE SAFETY AND PROFESSIONALISM?

To support professionalism in the workplace requires the pursuit of a safety culture, which cannot be achieved solely based on the courage of team members—there needs to be a plan that is supported by the right *people*, *organization*, and *learning culture* (**Fig. 5**). While a detailed discussion of this infrastructure is beyond the scope of

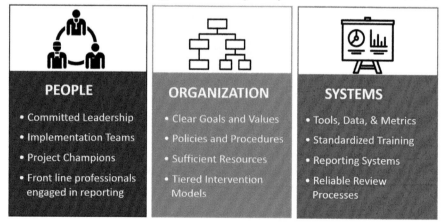

Accountability and High Reliability Require an Infrastructure

PEOPLE	ORGANIZATION	SYSTEMS
• Committed Leadership	• Clear Goals and Values	• Tools, Data, & Metrics
• Implementation Teams	• Policies and Procedures	• Standardized Training
• Project Champions	• Sufficient Resources	• Reporting Systems
• Front line professionals engaged in reporting	• Tiered Intervention Models	• Reliable Review Processes

Fig. 5. Structural elements for promoting accountability and high reliability. People, organization, and systems are the building blocks for supporting professional accountability and allow for progress toward high reliability. Leadership, infrastructure, and metrics/tools are critical. *From* Joint Commission Resources.

this article, understanding the rudiments can assist readers in considering what actions they can take in their own practice, hospital, or system.

An example of a tiered intervention model to provide feedback on any kind of performance is the Vanderbilt Promoting Professionalism Pyramid (**Fig. 6**), which has been successfully used to promote hand hygiene, promote vaccine administration, and address clinical team members who model disrespect.[27–29] The pyramid is based on the knowledge that the vast majority of clinical team members are committed to doing the right thing. That said, medicine is complex and stressful, and all professionals are subject to an occasional lapse in performance. If, for example, a Dr Scalpelle exhibits behavior that intimidates other members of the team or he fails to participate in the time-out process, a team member is encouraged to speak up in the moment or share observations through a safety reporting system.

Reports are reviewed in a timely manner and (if not mandated for investigation due to an assertion of physical contact, sexual boundary violation, or discrimination, as represented by the orange triangle in the lower right corner of **Fig 6**)[27] are dispatched to a peer messenger for delivery. The peer is trained to share the report with Dr

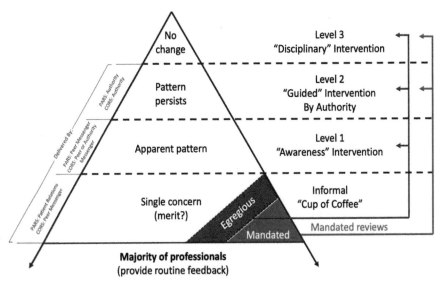

Fig. 6. Promoting professionalism pyramid. The pyramid illustrates a tiered intervention approach that supports the pursuit of professional accountability. Recorded reports are reviewed and can be shared in a respectful, nondirective fashion during an informal conversation such as one might have with a colleague over a cup of coffee.

- When patterns of persistent concerns emerge, a peer-delivered Level 1 Awareness Intervention, with local and national peer comparisons, is performed.
- Clinicians who are unable or unwilling to respond are escalated to Guided Interventions by Authority (Level 2), which includes authority figure (eg, department chair, Chief Medical Officer).
- A very small number may not respond and are elevated to Level 3 disciplinary action as defined by organizational policies, bylaws, contracts, or other governing documents. (*Adapted with permission from* Hickson GB, Pichert JW, Webb LE, Gabbe SG. A complementary approach to promoting professionalism: Identifying, measuring, and addressing unprofessional behaviors. Acad. Med. 2007 Nov; 82 (11): 1040-1048.)

Scalpelle in a nonjudgmental, nondirective meeting, while sharing a cup of coffee. Approximately, 70% of individuals will respond without other reports (over a 3-year audit period).[30] If a pattern emerges (less than 5% of clinicians), an *Awareness Intervention* (Level 1) is delivered. Individuals who are unwilling to change or unable to do so (eg, those whose complaints arise from neurocognitive impairment[31]) are escalated to a *Guided Interventions by Authority* (Level 2), with a written corrective plan by the department chair or Chief Medical Officer (less than 1.5% of clinicians). Rarely, a *Disciplinary Intervention* (Level 3) is needed, invoking organizational policies, bylaws, contracts, or other governing documents.

When single incidents are not addressed, patterns are more likely to emerge, sometimes rippling through the organization.[12,32–36] Unprofessional behavior compromises communication, teamwork, and trust, negatively impacting patient care and safety. These behaviors may have adverse effects for nurses, residents, and patients, who are more likely to suffer preventable medical or surgical complications.[10,37,38] Maintaining professional standards is only possible when structures are in place that support an organized approach to delivering the firsthand accounts of patients and coworkers in a timely fashion, thereby reinforcing a culture of safety. Leaders must hold everyone accountable equally; employ and utilize reporting systems; and invest necessary resources to individuals and teams to build and maintain the efforts.

Fig. 7 illustrates variation in how individuals may reflect and adjust their performance based on feedback. Serving coffee or making someone aware that there appears to be a pattern of unprofessional behavior is about calling on professionals to reflect and self-regulate. In the example of the blue line, the clinician alters her behavior after meeting with a respectful colleague over coffee. She thereby rejoins coworkers in resuming professional behaviors that reinforce patient safety and the well-being of the team. The green line, in contrast, depicts a clinician who

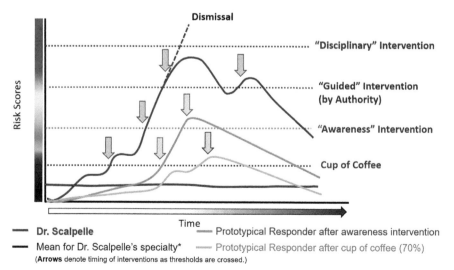

Professional Risk Profiles Over Time

Fig. 7. Professional response to tiered interventions. The hypothetical profiles of clinicians depicted by red, green, and blue lines illustrate how individuals may differ in their responses to feedback provided over coffee or, if required, to subsequent escalating interventions.

does not respond when coffee is served. By his behavior and performance, he exhibits ongoing slips and lapses of self-regulation that separate him from his professional colleagues; however, in response to the awareness intervention, this clinician returns to accepted norms and rejoins colleagues.

Sometimes, albeit rarely, individuals graduate to higher levels of interventions. Dr Scalpelle (red line) is recalcitrant and proceeds to a guided intervention after responding to neither coffee nor an *Awareness* Intervention. The depiction foreshadows professional lapses—and interventions in response to them—that unfold in Parts 2 and 3 of this series. If Dr Scalpelle eventually responds to the interventions (solid line), he rejoins the professional community; in contrast, if he does not, he is among the small number of professionals who requires a disciplinary intervention, and possibly even restriction of privileges, dismissal, or nonrenewal (depicted by dotted line). The goal for all clinicians requiring these interventions is to help them rejoin their professional colleagues, and the pyramid supports them in doing so. Barring organic illness, such as brain tumor, neurodegenerative disease, or cognitive decline, it is their choice. Best practices for referring clinicians for help are shown in **Fig. 8**.

IS PROMOTING PROFESSIONALISM SOUND BUSINESS PRACTICE?

Medical malpractice claims and legal costs account for a substantial portion of expenditures across health care organizations. In recent years, the trend has been one of increasing severity of claims, corresponding to higher payouts.[39–43] Many members of the health care community—particularly physicians and surgeons—have a certain fatalism about malpractice claims—regarding them as inevitable and therefore "the

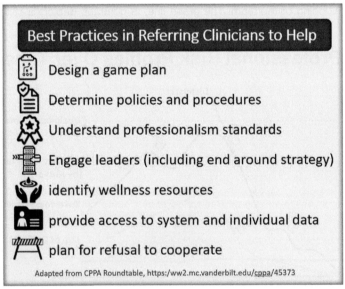

Fig. 8. Referring clinicians for professional assistance.*(Adapted from* CCPA Roundtable https://nam11.safelinks.protection.outlook.com/?url=https%3A%2F%2Fww2.mc. vanderbilt.edu%2Fcppa%2F45373&data=04%7C01%7Cj.surendrakumar%40elsevier.com% 7Ce2dd426f9cb2421e8fa308d96657f271%7C9274ee3f94254109a27f9fb15c10675d%7C0% 7C0%7C637653351109775840%7CUnknown%7CTWFpbGZsb3d8eyJWIjoiMC4wLjAwMDAiL CJQIjoiV2luMzIiLCJBTiI6Ik1haWwiLCJXVCI6Mn0%3D%7C1000&sdata=z4fY5lQYuL3r% 2FqByrMwrB4%2FXj7ZNZj298GMc6FrB7WI%3D&reserved=0.)

cost of doing business." To others, litigation is like lightning, striking with tremendous destructive force, without reason or any means of prevention. The data tell a different story, however. Studies into why patients and families pursue claims do not show arbitrariness but rather reveal recurring themes—including concerns around the care delivered, concerns about inadequacy of the explanation for what happened, or concerns for similar incidents happening again.[23,44–46]

The data are clear that some clinicians are litigation lightning rods, and adverse surgical outcomes often can be traced to teams disrupted by unprofessional behavior.[24,25] The risk of adverse events spikes when the surgical team neglects to do a timeout, fails to protect the surgical field, or deviates from best practice—often to avoid criticism or to appease a volatile team member. When a patient gets an infection, the prior disclosure of this risk during informed consent may matter little to the patient who has been shown disrespect at any point during his or her care; suspicion only rises when a disrespected team members intimates to the family that they are not surprised, because the surgeon's patients "seem" to have more infections. Tiered interventions are highly effective in addressing unprofessional behavior, with very few physicians reaching the top tier of disciplinary interventions.

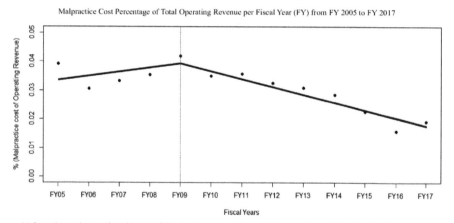

Malpractice savings reduced by 50% following implementation of Risk Reduction Initiative (vertical line)

Fig. 9. Reduction in malpractice costs associated with tiered interventions. Malpractice expenditures decreased by 50% over a 7-year period after implementation of a tiered strategy. (*From* Diraviam et. al., Physician Engagement in Malpractice Risk Reduction: A UPHS Case Study, The Joint Commission Journal on Quality and Patient Safety, Volume 44, Issue 10, 2018,Pages 605-612. Available at: https://nam11.safelinks.protection.outlook.com/?url=https%3A%2F%2Fdoi.org%2F10.1016%2Fj.jcjq.2018.03.009&data=04%7C01%7Cj.surendrakumar%40elsevier.com%7Ce2dd426f9cb2421e8fa308d96657f271%7C9274ee3f94254109a27f9fb15c10675d%7C0%7C0%7C637653351109775840%7CUnknown%7CTWFpbGZsb3d8eyJWIjoiMC4wLjAwMDAiLCJQIjoiV2luMzIiLCJBTiI6Ik1haWwiLCJXVCI6Mn0%3D%7C1000&sdata=hrqc%2BDd8X%2FQ5rbPEy0pBRl%2Bh6%2BqUZls93MIHl0k2jJM%3D&reserved=0.(https://nam11.safelinks.protection.outlook.com/?url=https%3A%2F%2Fwww.sciencedirect.com%2Fscience%2Farticle%2Fpii%2FS1553725017304749&data=04%7C01%7Cj.surendrakumar%40elsevier.com%7Ce2dd426f9cb2421e8fa308d96657f271%7C9274ee3f94254109a27f9fb15c10675d%7C0%7C0%7C637653351109785837%7CUnknown%7CTWFpbGZsb3d8eyJWIjoiMC4wLjAwMDAiLCJQIjoiV2luMzIiLCJBTiI6Ik1haWwiLCJXVCI6Mn0%3D%7C1000&sdata=%2F%2B8O8pBAM8oRzILZ9m9tyllol%2B9itBXFbCqxXO58Euw%3D&reserved=0)

In response to a high number of malpractice claims and payouts, the University of Pennsylvania Health System (UPHS) implemented a risk reduction strategy that incorporated the Vanderbilt Patient Advocacy Reporting System (PARS)[26] including the tiered intervention model, and actively engaged physicians in addressing unprofessional behaviors.[47] Using data captured by their office of patient relations and coded and aggregated by the Vanderbilt team, the institution identified their physicians at high malpractice claims risk. Physicians at 1.5 to 2 standard deviations above the mean for their specialty underwent tiered professionalism interventions, beginning with awareness and, only if required, escalation to authority-based interventions.[28] The strategy resulted in halving of malpractice costs, from approximately 4% to 2% of total UPHS patient service revenues during the 7-year study period (**Fig. 9**).

BRINGING IT ALL TOGETHER: PURSUIT OF HIGH RELIABILITY

Worldwide, innumerable patients suffer injuries, permanent disabilities, and death from patient safety events that might have been prevented. While the modern safety movement has ushered in prodigious efforts to encourage improvement, the evidence of progress remains limited. Is care measurably safer than it was two decades ago? The answer is likely mixed. Much more is understood about medical errors,[48] and there is heightened awareness of human factors engineering and root cause analysis and actions[49] — areas explored in Part 2. Nonetheless, reluctance or inability to hold individuals accountable may partially explain the challenge of achieving transformative change in health care. System considerations are important, but limiting case reviews solely to system issues can dilute personal accountability — leaving the door open for a Dr Scalpelle to walk in and immediately impact individual and team performance; discounting the importance of individual behaviors may make it nearly impossible to identify contributing factors that led to a tragic event.[50]

The practice of medicine is inherently dangerous, and the ideal is "failure-free operation... safe, effective, patient-centered, timely, efficient, and equitable." The

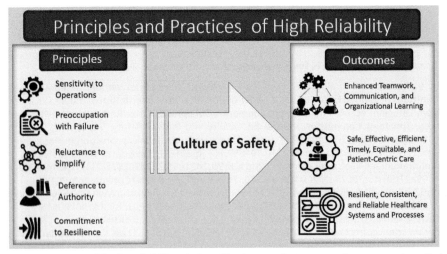

Fig. 10. Pursuit of high reliability. Safe, effective, patient-centered care requires that embracing the principles of high-reliability organizations, which involve a combination of curiosity, rigor, and resilience in correcting sources of failure and promoting optimal teamwork.

characteristics of high-reliability organizations are shown in **Fig. 10**. In academic discussions of high reliability, the emphasis is often on the hard-headed perseverance necessary to drill down to the proximate cause of failure and to eradicate it, but in practice, there is another ingredient that is critical—curiosity. Without a deep sense of inquisitiveness, one does not trouble to turn over the stones necessary to uncover the cause of unexpected outcomes. Behaviors that undermine safety can evade detection far more readily than clinical metrics or laboratory values, especially when team members hesitate to speak up for whatever reason.

The pursuit of high reliability requires alignment of vision, goals, and core values. Leadership is indispensable in this journey,[51] and a safety culture must afford psychological safety and trust. Health care professionals have a solemn duty to provide the highest quality care possible, which requires reinforcing accountability across *all* health care professionals. Historically, this principle of consistent accountability has not always been honored. Casting a blind eye on unprofessional behavior shields clinicians who threaten teams and outcomes.[52] Most of the time, the team manages to achieve a heroic rescue—often by a nurse, anesthesiologist, or learner who has the courage to speak up—but sometimes nobody speaks up, and the journey toward high reliability is derailed. Hope is never a plan. That is why an infrastructure is needed.

Team training and champions play an important role in promoting a safety culture. Medical team training improves outcomes of surgical care, reducing surgical mortality in a large, multi-institutional study.[53] A professional champion can be tremendously valuable for developing and sustaining plans. The champion has influence by virtue of energy, a sense of humor, and an ability to promote change. Effective project champions have capital within the organization, and they are willing to use their influence to benefit the project. They also may be nontraditional or entrepreneurial, going well beyond expected and traditional job responsibilities.[54] Examples of these nontraditional side qualities are depicted in **Fig. 11**. Champions can be instrumental in efforts to balance individual accountability with system-based effforts.[50]

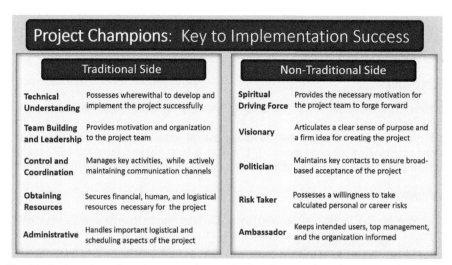

Fig. 11. Project champions. In supporting professionalism, project champions play a vital role and often differ from conventional project managers in having an orientation toward a nontraditional side.

Some of the questions that frontline professionals and leaders should contemplate are as follows:

- What people or systems within your organization are contributing to a culture of silence or transparency?
- How can reporting be encouraged and become the norm?
- Is there a defined and fair plan to address disrespectful/unprofessional behavior, including a plan to escalate as needed?
- Is the plan sturdy enough to withstand pressures, such that leaders will not blink because of the perceived special value of a clinician?

Reporting systems coupled with a tiered accountability plan support the institutional journey to professional behavior. The *people* are critical for leadership commitment; the *organization* supports the values, policies, and interventions; and the *system* allows for data capture and structures to sustain the efforts. Only when these elements are integrated can transformative change be achieved. The culture of reporting is critical, as is response to these reports. A first-rate cup of coffee is delivered hot—ideally within 48 hours so that professionals receive swift, timely feedback—and it is offered in a spirit of collegiality. Coffee served cold, stale, or acidic is far less effective. The worst cup of coffee, however, is the cup not served at all.

SUMMARY

Patients place their lives in the hands of their health care team, and every member of that team is beholden to professionalism in service of patients' best interest. The pursuit of high reliability is predicated on not only individual technical and cognitive competence but also the self-regulation, self-awareness, respect, and effective communication necessary for effective teamwork. The Promoting Professionalism Pyramid is a proven framework for identifying areas in need of improvement and then addressing unprofessional behaviors through tiered interventions. Successful implementation requires leadership commitment, use of consistent standards, and investment in necessary infrastructure. These efforts translate into improved patient experience, enhanced safety, and reduced risk of litigation. Despite best efforts, however, medicine is not entirely predictable; the next article in this series, *Communication and Transparency (Part 2),* offers a principled and comprehensive approach for responding to patient harm.

DISCLOSURES

Dr Hickson is an employee of Vanderbilt University Medical Center; is a member of Medtronic's speakers bureau. He receives royalties from Cognitive Institute; and has received payment for the development of educational presentations from numerous health care institutions. Dr Hickson is also a member of the USC Health System Board and Vice Chair of the Institute for Healthcare Improvement (IHI) Board.

REFERENCES

1. Lencione P. The advantage: why organizational health trumps everything else in business. San Francisco: Jossey- Bass, HB Printing; 2012.
2. Yeoman G, Furlong P, Seres M, et al. Defining patient centricity with patients for patients and caregivers: a collaborative endeavour. BMJ Innov 2017;3(2):76–83.
3. Institute TB. The declaration for human experience. 2021. Available at: https://transformhx.org/. Accessed July 5, 2021.

4. Standiford T, Shuman AG, Fessell D, et al. Upholding the tripartite mission in times of crisis: purpose and perseverance in the COVID-19 pandemic. Otolaryngol Head Neck Surg 2020;163(1):54–9.

5. Brenner MJ. A piece of my mind. Collateral damage. JAMA 2009;301(16): 1637–8.

6. Boothman RC, Blackwell AC, Campbell DA Jr, et al. A better approach to medical malpractice claims? The University of Michigan experience. J Health Life Sci Law 2009;2(2):125–59.

7. Kirch DG. Culture and the courage to change. AAMC President's address, presented at the 118th annual meeting of the association of American medical colleges, Washington, DC, November 4, 2010.

8. Martinez W, Hickson GB, Miller BM, et al. Role-modeling and medical error disclosure: a national survey of trainees. Acad Med 2014;89(3):482–9.

9. Sydor DT, Bould MD, Naik VN, et al. Challenging authority during a life-threatening crisis: the effect of operating theatre hierarchy. Br J Anaesth 2013; 110(3):463–71.

10. Raemer DB, Kolbe M, Minehart RD, et al. Improving anesthesiologists' ability to speak up in the operating room: a randomized controlled experiment of a simulation-based intervention and a qualitative analysis of hurdles and enablers. Acad Med 2016;91(4):530–9.

11. Weinger MB, Banerjee A, Burden AR, et al. Simulation-based assessment of the management of critical events by board-certified anesthesiologists. Anesthesiology 2017;127(3):475–89.

12. Gaba DM, Howard SK, Jump B. Production pressure in the work environment. California anesthesiologists' attitudes and experiences. Anesthesiology 1994; 81(2):488–500.

13. Gaba DM, Howard SK, Flanagan B, et al. Assessment of clinical performance during simulated crises using both technical and behavioral ratings. Anesthesiology 1998;89(1):8–18.

14. Edmonson AC. Teamwork on the fly: how to master the new art of teaming. 2012. Available at: https://workforcesummit.ucsf.edu/sites/g/files/tkssra1166/f/Edmondson_Teaming_on_the_Fly.pdf. Accessed July 8, 2021.

15. Halbesleben JR, Rathert C. Linking physician burnout and patient outcomes: exploring the dyadic relationship between physicians and patients. Health Care Manage Rev 2008;33(1):29–39.

16. Ahmadmehrabi S, Farlow JL, Wamkpah NS, et al. New age mentoring and disruptive innovation-navigating the uncharted with vision, purpose, and equity. JAMA Otolaryngol Head Neck Surg 2021;147(4):389–94.

17. Prince ADP, Green AR, Brown DJ, et al. The clarion call of the COVID-19 pandemic: how medical education can mitigate racial and ethnic disparities. Acad Med 2021.

18. Ofri D. When we do harm: a doctor confronts medical error. Boston: Beacon Press; 2020.

19. Nurses AAoC-C. Silence kills. Nursing 2005;35(4):33. Available at: https://journals.lww.com/nursing/fulltext/2005/04000/_silence_kills_.27.aspx.

20. Google. Google's Project Aristotle - re:Work. Available at: https://rework.withgoogle.com/guides/understanding-team-effectiveness/steps/introduction/. Accessed June 29, 2021.

21. Lencione P. The five dysfunctions of a team: a leadership fable. San Francisco: Jossey-Bass; 2002.

22. Edmonson AC, Lei Z. Psychological safety: The history, renaissance, and future of an interpersonal construct. Annu Rev Organ Psychol Organ Behav 2014; 1(1):23–43.
23. Hickson GB, Federspiel CF, Pichert JW, et al. Patient complaints and malpractice risk. JAMA 2002;287(22):2951–7.
24. Cooper WO, Guillamondegui O, Hines OJ, et al. Use of unsolicited patient observations to identify surgeons with increased risk for postoperative complications. JAMA Surg 2017;152(6):522–9.
25. Cooper WO, Spain DA, Guillamondegui O, et al. Association of coworker reports about unprofessional behavior by surgeons with surgical complications in their patients. JAMA Surg 2019;154(9):828–34.
26. Nassiri AM, Pichert JW, Domenico HJ, et al. Unsolicited patient complaints among otolaryngologists. Otolaryngol Head Neck Surg 2019;160(5):810–7.
27. Hickson GB, Pichert JW, Webb LE, et al. A complementary approach to promoting professionalism: identifying, measuring, and addressing unprofessional behaviors. Acad Med 2007;82(11):1040–8.
28. Pichert JW, Moore IN, Karrass J, et al. An intervention model that promotes accountability: peer messengers and patient/family complaints. Jt Comm J Qual Patient Saf 2013;39(10):435–46.
29. Talbot TR, Johnson JG, Fergus C, et al. Sustained improvement in hand hygiene adherence: utilizing shared accountability and financial incentives. Infect Control Hosp Epidemiol 2013;34(11):1129–36.
30. Webb LE, Dmochowski RR, Moore IN, et al. Using coworker observations to promote accountability for disrespectful and unsafe behaviors by physicians and advanced practice professionals. Jt Comm J Qual Patient Saf 2016;42(4):149–64.
31. Cooper WO, Martinez W, Domenico HJ, et al. Unsolicited patient complaints identify physicians with evidence of neurocognitive disorders. Am J Geriatr Psychiatry 2018;26(9):927–36.
32. Sessler DI, Khanna AK. Perioperative myocardial injury and the contribution of hypotension. Intensive Care Med 2018;44(6):811–22.
33. Lingard L, Reznick R, Espin S, et al. Team communications in the operating room: talk patterns, sites of tension, and implications for novices. Acad Med 2002;77(3):232–7.
34. Leape LL, Brennan TA, Laird N, et al. The nature of adverse events in hospitalized patients. Results of the Harvard Medical Practice Study II. N Engl J Med 1991; 324(6):377–84.
35. Grade MM, Tamboli MK, Bereknyei Merrell S, et al. Attending surgeons differ from other team members in their perceptions of operating room communication. J Surg Res 2019;235:105–12.
36. Belyansky I, Martin TR, Prabhu AS, et al. Poor resident-attending intraoperative communication may compromise patient safety. J Surg Res 2011;171(2):386–94.
37. Pian-Smith MC, Simon R, Minehart RD, et al. Teaching residents the two-challenge rule: a simulation-based approach to improve education and patient safety. Simul Healthc 2009;4(2):84–91.
38. Friedman Z, Hayter MA, Everett TC, et al. Power and conflict: the effect of a superior's interpersonal behaviour on trainees' ability to challenge authority during a simulated airway emergency. Anaesthesia 2015;70(10):1119–29.
39. New CRICO Comparative Benchmarking System report indicates claim frequency down; claim severity, management costs up. Medical Liability Monitor March 2019;44(3):1–7. Available at. https://www.rmf.harvard.edu/about-crico/media/in-the-news/news/2019/march/new-crico-comparative-benchmarking-system-report.

40. Malpractice claims Frequency holding steady while severity increases. 2020. Available at: *https://www.claimsjournal.com/news/national/2020/10/15/299950. htm.* Accessed July 5, 2021.
41. Medical professional liability market facing difficult times. Insurance Journal 2021. Available at: https://www.insurancejournal.com/news/national/2021/05/13/ 613756.htm. Accessed July 5, 2021.
42. Burke AH, Lambrecht A, Patel A, et al. A call for action: insights from a decade of malpractice claims. 2020. Available at: https://www.coverys.com/PDFs/call-for-action-decade-of-malpractice-claims.aspx. Accessed July 5, 2021.
43. Salter A. The state of the medical malpractice market. 2020. Available at: https:// geneseeins.com/the-state-of-the-medical-malpractice-market/. Accessed July 5, 2021.
44. Hickson GB, Clayton EW, Entman SS, et al. Obstetricians' prior malpractice experience and patients' satisfaction with care. JAMA 1994;272(20):1583–7.
45. Hickson GB, Clayton EW, Githens PB, et al. Factors that prompted families to file medical malpractice claims following perinatal injuries. JAMA 1992;267(10): 1359–63.
46. Hickson GB, Jenkins AD. Identifying and addressing communication failures as a means of reducing unnecessary malpractice claims. N C Med J 2007;68(5): 362–4.
47. Greco PJ, Eisenberg JM. Changing physicians' practices. N Engl J Med 1993; 329(17):1271–3.
48. Brenner MJ, Chang CWD, Boss EF, et al. Patient safety/quality improvement primer, part I: what PS/QI means to your otolaryngology practice. Otolaryngol Head Neck Surg 2018;159(1):3–10.
49. Balakrishnan K, Brenner MJ, Gosbee JW, et al. Patient safety/quality improvement primer, part II: prevention of harm through root cause analysis and action (RCA(2)). Otolaryngol Head Neck Surg 2019;161(6):911–21.
50. Hickson GB, Moore IN, Pichert JW, et al. Balancing systems and individual accountability in a safety culture. Chapter 1. In: Berman S, editor. From front office to front line. Essential issues for healthcare leaders. 2nd edition. Oakbrook Terrace, IL: Joint Commission Resources; 2012. p. 1–36.
51. Boothman RCH GB. Time to rethink physician leadership training?. In: Physician leadership journal. Atlanta, GA: American Association for Physician Leadership; 2021. p. 41–6.
52. Felps WM TR, Byington E. How, when, and why bad apples spoil the barrel: negative group members and dysfunctional groups. Res Organ Behav 2006; 27:175–222.
53. Neily J, Mills PD, Young-Xu Y, et al. Association between implementation of a medical team training program and surgical mortality. JAMA 2010;304(15): 1693–700.
54. Pinto JK, Slevin DP. The project champion: key to implementation success. Proj Manag J 1989;20(4):15–20.

Honesty and Transparency, Indispensable to the Clinical Mission—Part II

How Communication and Resolution Programs Promote Patient Safety and Trust

Michael J. Brenner, MD[a,b,]*, Gerald B. Hickson, MD[c,d],
Cynda Hylton Rushton, PhD, MSN, RN[e,f,g],
Mark E.P. Prince, MD, FRCS(C)[a,h], Carol R. Bradford, MD, MS[a,i,j],
Richard C. Boothman, JD[k,l,m]

KEYWORDS

- Patient safety • Adverse events • Communication and resolution program • Honesty
- Transparency • Quality improvement • Medical errors

KEY POINTS

- After an adverse event, the traumatizing effects on patients, families, and health care professionals are magnified by a deny-and-defend response, which deepens wounds, impedes improvement, and erodes trust.
- To counteract decades of blind deference to the legal and insurance professions, leadership must insist on a response to patients harmed by their care that aligns with and serves the clinical mission.

Continued

---

[a] Department of Otolaryngology–Head & Neck Surgery, University of Michigan Medical School, Ann Arbor; [b] GTC Quality Improvement Collaborative, Durham, NC, USA; [c] Center for Patient and Professional Advocacy, Vanderbilt University Medical Center, Nashville, TN, USA; [d] Center for Quality, Safety and Risk Prevention, Vanderbilt University Medical Center, Nashville, TN, USA; [e] Johns Hopkins University School of Nursing, Baltimore, MD, USA; [f] Department of Pediatrics, Johns Hopkins University School of Medicine, Baltimore, MD, USA; [g] Berman Institute of Bioethics, Johns Hopkins University School of Medicine, Baltimore, MD, USA; [h] Rogel Cancer Center, University of Michigan Medical School, Ann Arbor, MI, USA; [i] The College of Medicine and James Cancer Hospital and Solove Research Institute; [j] Department of Otolaryngology–Head and Neck Surgery, The Ohio State University Wexner Medical Center, Columbus; [k] Boothman Consulting Group, LLC, Ann Arbor, MI, USA; [l] Department of Surgery, University of Michigan Medical School, Ann Arbor; [m] Center for Patient and Professional Advocacy, Vanderbilt University Medical Center, Nashville, TN, USA
* Corresponding author. Department of Otolaryngology-Head & Neck Surgery, University of Michigan School of Medicine, 1500 East Medical Center Drive SPC 5312, 1904 Taubman Center, Ann Arbor, MI 48109-5312.
E-mail address: mbren@med.umich.edu

Otolaryngol Clin N Am 55 (2022) 63–82
https://doi.org/10.1016/j.otc.2021.07.018
0030-6665/22/© 2021 Elsevier Inc. All rights reserved.

oto.theclinics.com

Continued

- Communication and resolution programs provide a principled, comprehensive, and systematic approach for responding transparently and empathically to unintended patient harm, ameliorating the harm to patients and clinical staff while prioritizing rapid clinical improvement and health care professional well-being.
- In addition to improving care and delivering swifter justice, experience to date with communication and resolution programs suggests a potential decrease in legal expenditures and turnover among health care professionals.

A lack of transparency results in distrust and a deep sense of insecurity.
—*Dalai Lama*

INTRODUCTION

Health care is fraught with risk of unintentional harm, and even with our best efforts, adverse events may occur during patient care. Clinicians require a cohesive framework for responding to patient harm in a principled and proactive manner. Part 1 of this series opened with a case that illustrated the role of professionalism in promoting patient safety. The anesthesia resident, Dr Lerner, was initiating a sedation anesthetic for a nasal skin cancer reconstruction after Mohs excision. The surgery attending, Dr Scalpelle, pushed for deeper sedation, leading to apnea with recovery—a near miss.

The patient is unharmed, but the team experiences an erosion of trust. Not only has the power dynamic between Drs Scalpelle and Lerner disrupted effective teamwork, but the team members are jarred by how Dr Resedent, the surgical resident, pushed aside Nurse Corage to perform a jaw thrust when restoring oxygenation—mirroring Dr Scalpelle's negative role modeling. Thoughtfully capturing and responding to near misses and unintended clinical outcomes is essential to developing a culture marked by continual improvement and enhanced patient safety. The case discussion of professionalism in Part 1 sets the stage for discussing the second pillar, communication and transparency, as depicted in **Fig. 1**.

The case further unfolds in Part 2 of this trilogy, with an adverse event that profoundly affects the patient, family, and the entire health care team. This article addresses recognizing, reporting, and responding to a harm event—addressing harm with the patient and family in a way that conveys empathy and enhances safety across the continuum of care. We consider how societal and cultural forces, as well as human nature, powerfully contribute to a tendency to become defensive; shame and fear can be greatly amplified amid fears of litigation.

To rise to this challenge, communication and resolution programs provide a principled, comprehensive, and systematic approach for responding.[1,2] This approach sidesteps many of the deleterious effects of traditional legal approaches and advances clinical accountability and patient safety. Normalizing honesty and transparency after unintended outcomes—and doing so consistently, patient by patient—quickly builds an accountable culture that prioritizes patient safety. This emphasis on safety drives process improvements, engenders trust, and fosters health care team resilience in service of the organizational mission of patient centricity.

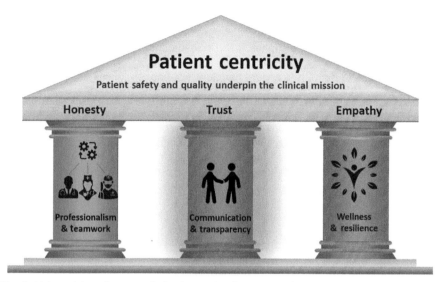

Fig. 1. Values-driven framework for improving honesty and transparency around adverse events. The core values of honesty, trust, and empathy are the basis for delivering safe, high quality care. Professionalism and teamwork (part 1) introduced tiered interventions that promote professional accountability. Communication and transparency (part 2) offers a principled approach for responding to patient harm. Wellness and resilience (part 3) explores burnout moral injury, and leadership solutions to restore joy in work and resilience.

CASE STUDY (CONTINUED FROM PART 1)

Dr Propofal, the anesthesia attending, arrives to find Dr Lerner looking visibly shaken, but she says nothing, recalling Dr Scalpelle's many prior fractious interactions with other learners. Ms Corage, an experienced operating room nurse who usually works in obstetrics and gynecology cases, asks Dr Scalpelle for direction on how the surgical site should prepped. Dr Scalpelle, visibly annoyed by question, rolls his eyes and, says sarcastically, "Surprise me." Nurse Corage begins cleansing the surgical field with an alcohol-based skin preparation as Drs Scalpelle and Resedent leave the room to scrub. When they return, Ms Corage voices a concern—as she prepped the site, the wound had started bleeding briskly. Dr Scalpelle sighs theatrically, directs Dr Resedent to hold pressure on the site, and asks in an irritated tone of voice, "Are we ready to get started NOW?"

The scrub technologist interjects, "First, we need to do a time-out." Avoiding eye contact with Dr Scalpelle, he hurries through the surgical safety checklist, bypassing the fire safety questions on cue from Dr Scalpelle to move things along. Dr Resedent lifts the gauze away, and brisk bleeding ensues. Dr Scalpelle reflexively takes hold of the electrocautery and directs it to the bleeding site. Suddenly, a yellow halo envelops the field, and the scrub technologist shouts "FIRE!!" Dr Lerner turns the oxygen off, and the fire is promptly extinguished. The patient lets out an agonized cry, abruptly roused by the searing heat, but confused and disoriented. The skin is burned, with eschar tracking ominously back to the nares and lips.

Reflect on a few questions:

- How should the open surgical site be handled? Should the airway be evaluated?
- Who should discuss the incident and plan with the family? What should be shared?

- What were the patterns of communication and behaviors that contributed to the harm?
- Are there any barriers to honesty and transparency? If so, how can these be overcome?
- What needs to happen to ensure this does not happen again?

The burns in proximity to the nasal and oral passages raise the specter of an airway injury. The team wants to evaluate the airway, but they have not obtained consent for these additional procedures. Drs Scalpelle and Propofal get the Office of General Counsel on the phone, and they are instructed to disclose only the facts—that a fire occurred and confirmed injuries. And do not discuss why the harm occurred, do not mention unconfirmed or possible ongoing harm, and do not admit any fault. Dr Propofal and Dr Scalpelle accept these directives and briefly explain to the stunned family that there was an operating room fire, that they have aborted the case, but that additional steps will be necessary in the operating room to evaluate the patient's airway. Left with no alternatives, they give consent for endoscopy.

Laryngoscopy and bronchoscopy show hyperemia of the nasal passages, mouth, and upper aerodigestive tract, with focal eschar near the nares. In response to the family's questions about how this happened, Dr Scalpelle brusquely notes that they need to get back to the operating room; Dr Propofal murmurs that these events are rare but happen, that they will need to investigate and will address their questions later. Risk management is notified. As he leaves the family, Dr Scalpelle growls, "I'm sure we'll all get sued for this one." The reconstruction is completed 2 days later.

UNDERSTANDING HARM

"Harm" in health care is a peculiar term; almost every invasive procedure causes a measure of injury or risk to tissues, yet it is only labeled harm after the fact, when an unexpected injury results. Surgically opening an operative site invariably severs small nerves and blood vessels, exposes tissues to infection, causes bleeding and reparative scar tissue, and risks inadvertent trauma to critical adjacent structures. None of these consequences of surgery are regarded as "patient harm"—depending on the clinical outcome. This distinction highlights the nuanced language of surgery and the privilege of performing it. The relationship between adverse events, errors, and patient harm is a relative one and significantly colors patients' perceptions (**Fig. 2**), not to mention the impact, ignored for decades, on health care professionals.[3]

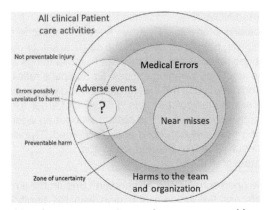

Fig. 2. Interrelationship of errors, near misses, adverse events, and harm.

When patients are harmed by their care, concerns fan out in all directions.[4] The patient must contend with the immediate and myriad consequences of that harm, which infiltrate most every facet of their lives: new short-term physical and emotional needs, the need to adjust to a new longer term reality, and the specter of future consequences including often-crippling financial costs, employment disruption, new financial demands, or even a loss of independence. Few families avoid the ripples from harm to a loved one. The raw realities of such experiences are harrowing in any situation, but they are greatly magnified by the realization, in many instances, that such harm was preventable. Patients and their families have complex and multifaceted needs after harm occurs (**Fig. 3**).

Apart from the daunting new challenges awaiting the patient and family, consider the impact on health care professionals, who experience their own trauma as they find themselves wound up in the unexpected patient outcome. The powerful mix of emotions may express themselves in difficulty concentrating, distraction, irritability, or self-isolation. Immediately after such episodes, professionals seldom have the luxury of a time-out to process what happened; they are expected to treat the next patients lined up in clinic or the operating room. Meanwhile, they have to figure out how to contend with the demands on time and energy to respond to the patient safety event and enlist necessary expertise. Affected members of the health care team may also struggle with complex questions of what happened and why, with incomplete clarity on the outcome or what stakeholders, such as leadership or legal counsel to notify and the implications of making those calls. Part 3 in this series provides an in-depth examination of strategies to address the needs of clinician.

After patient harm comes to light, there is another critically important stakeholder whose interests have rarely been treated as urgent—patients who have not been harmed yet. If harm happened to one, it could happen to others. How a new team member is received reflects the safety culture. Consider the reception of Nurse Corage—a highly trained nurse who has earned her stripes, but while working in another surgical discipline. Dr Scalpelle expects a team that knows the drill—his drill. What sort of welcome does Nurse Corage receive? Was she treated with respect? Was she empowered do her part? Was she provided psychological safety, so that she could speak up if something is not right? How did she feel when pushed aside by

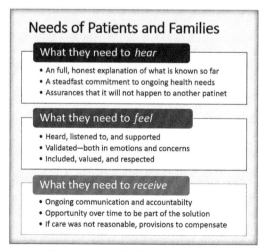

Fig. 3. Meeting the needs of patients and families after unintended harm.

Dr Resedent? How did Dr Scalpelle's sarcastic reply to her question about the preparation allow the selection of a flammable alcohol-based solution? And how did Dr Scalpelle's response to Nurse Corage's concerns about bleeding affect her readiness to alert the team to other concerns?

Several other questions relating to safety and risk or future fires also remain:

- Why were flammable alcohol-based preparation solutions available in an operating room where oxygen and cautery would be foreseeably needed?
- How did the pressure on the scrub technologist to rush through the surgical safety check list obscure awareness of fire risk or ways to mitigate such risk?
- What is the significance of Dr Propofal's passivity, remaining silent and unquestioning despite having repeatedly witnessed abrasive interactions or their aftermath?
- What is the likelihood that any of the operating room staff—including Nurse Corage—will ever complain about Dr Scalpelle after witnessing Dr Propofal's timidity?

Health care is inescapably dangerous; the risks cannot be controlled entirely, and patient harm, regardless of how it came about, should place everyone on notice that other patients are at risk—and it and should prompt measures that mitigate such risk. The speed and consistency with which patient harm is acknowledged, assessed, analyzed, and prevented matters. Inexplicably, health care's response to patient harm often disregards this inescapable fact.

Medicine happens in a moving stream of patient care, yet all too often, the fear of litigation arising from harm to an individual patient commands center stage—a fear that impedes evidence-based peer review, hampers important patient safety initiatives, and shelters challenged clinical practices and challenged clinical practitioners. It is a fear that has for decades prioritized the chance of financial loss from a single case at the risk of far more devastating human (and financial) consequences to other patients, other health care professionals and the organizations in which they work.

In the vignette, Dr Propofal tolerates behaviors that put patients and team members in harm's way. In doing so, Dr Propofal betrays her team, degrades team solidarity, and undermines safety. In a persistently hierarchical environment, Dr Propofal is a ranking member of the team and has a particular responsibility to those beneath her. The conspicuous assault on the psychological safety experienced by Dr Lerner, Nurse Corage, and the Scrub Technologist constrains their ability to raise concerns in the case and surely, for future cases. Much like removing the battery from a smoke detector will silence an uninvited chirp, the captain-of-the-ship tone created by Dr Scalpelle (and tacitly reinforced by Dr Propofal's silence) short circuits critical safeguards and greatly increases risk to the patient and to the team.

WHAT BARRIERS EXIST TO TRANSPARENCY AND EMPATHY?
Case (Continued)

Two weeks later, the patient remains upset, concerned about the skin sloughed from the burn and pain when opening his mouth. The family is convinced that the burns have worsened Mr Peyshent's breathing. Dr Resedent presents the case at the monthly departmental morbidity and mortality conference. Anxious and contrite, Dr Lerner is also present. Dr Propofal, continuing to abdicate her own responsibility to the team, is nowhere to be found. Dr Resedent nervously explains how she was party to a fire in the operating room and what has unfolded since. Dr Scalpelle stays silent, leaving Dr Resedent to explain. As other faculty begin to question what happened, a member of the general counsel's office interrupts the clinical presentation to remind the audience that events like these have myriad legal implications—including the risk of a large financial loss—and those in attendance must not to talk about the case with anyone.

For decades—some would say for more than a hundred years—the most common response to patient harm has been one of deny and defend, a term that graphically captures both the stonewalling ethos and legalistic context of this approach. Understanding its roots and its pervasiveness is necessary to improve current practices. Although it undoubtedly taps an ingrained human tendency to avoid perceived threats, deny and defend did not evolve naturally as a clinical response of health care professionals, nor was it inspired by foundational values of their clinical mission. Rather, it was instinctive to lawyers, insurance professionals, and risk managers trained to identify worst case scenarios with one overriding concern: the need to minimize the financial exposure from a potential medical malpractice claim.

Sadly short sighted, deny and defend not only subjugated patient-centered objectives to legal ones, but magnified the suffering of patients, families, and health care professionals. It inhibited clinical improvement and complicated any hope of professional self-policing. It is not normal for a health care professional to run away from an injured patient. It is not normal for a caregiver to deny an injured person compassion. It is not normal for professionals—who are trained to provide informed consent before delivering care—to withhold key information from someone later harmed in the course of that care. Given how deny and defend can cast a pall over the trusting relationship between clinicians and patients, we must make intentional and sustained efforts to reorient to our clinical mission.

Ironically, deny and defend sows the seeds for that which it is intended to avoid: litigation. The reasons patients sue doctors and health care organizations have been clear for decades: a desperate need for answers, a need for accountability, and a yearning for assurances that what happened to them will not happen to others.[5,6] Stonewalling is a particularly regrettable tactic because it deprives patients and families of the very connection and clarity needed for healing, leaving them no alternative but to retain an advocate.[7]

Plaintiff's lawyers working in medical malpractice almost invariably find that patients do not greet them with the goal of a financial windfall; instead, they ask lawyers to help them get answers, explanations, apologies, and protection for future patients. Constrained by courtroom limitations, plaintiffs' lawyers can only promise to fight for information and for a favorable jury verdict or settlement. Although very few patients are truly satisfied with this alternative, it is all they have historically been offered.

HOW DOES A LEGALISTIC FRAMING OF PATIENT HARM AFFECT HEALTH CARE PROFESSIONALS?

The deny-and-defend response to patient harm has a corrosive effect on the psyche of health care professionals. Physicians are routinely admonished not to say anything to the patient, not to show compassion lest it be misconstrued as an admission, not to admit to anything, not to talk to anyone other than their lawyer (most often a lawyer they did not choose), and to be circumspect about what they enter in the patient's record. Many believe they should not discuss the situation with their partners or spouses—and many would not anyway out of shame and fear. The advice has been to circle the wagons, keep their heads down, and wait for a lawsuit.

The threat of litigation, inherently demoralizing for clinicians, can interfere with the very processes most necessary to advance the clinical mission—peer review, quality improvement, and the pursuit of high reliability operations. Processes intended to serve patient safety often take a back seat, stymied or frozen by a legal process that did not evolve to meet the needs of patient. When these legal considerations drive a wedge between the patient and the health care team, all parties suffer. Legal remedies are a social expedient to resolve civil disputes, and they do little to address the real-time needs of patients requiring the ongoing care of health professionals. Because the legal profession neither has the same goals nor values as the clinical enterprise, being beholden to legal directives can cause frustration, cynicism, and distress.

Even if a strong defense case can be mounted, involved health care professionals must grapple with awareness that they may have caused harm, preventable or not. Health care is delivered amid a heady mix of the latest scientific knowledge, clinical outcomes data, and cutting-edge technology. After patient harm, lawyers evaluate the care retrospectively, when the outcome, always negative, is known. Answering the question, "Was the care reasonable?" requires recreating the surrounding circumstances—and often invention. Medical malpractice lawyers begin building a defense for an audience of jurors, in the theater of the courtroom. And none of the jurors will be a health care professional.

In his defense of Oklahoma City bombing suspect Terry Nichols, famed trial lawyer and law professor Michael Tigar observed, "An expert is someone who wasn't there when it happened, but who will, for a fee, gladly imagine what it must have been like." Lawyers on both sides easily find highly paid experts who will offer sworn testimony to a clinically unsophisticated audience of jurors. Frequently the expert testimonies are 180° apart, and the unsophisticated audience is expected to discern what is true and what is manufactured. Medicine has blindly deferred to professionals in insurance and law who were focused on goals unaligned with foundational principles of patient-centered care.

The following sections describe an alternative—communication and resolution programs, which offer a principled and comprehensive approach for responding to unintended harm. The overarching concept is that combining a commitment to honesty and transparency with the right infrastructure can serve patients and supplant deny-and-defend approaches. These programs can help individuals and institutions to overcome fear and protective reflexes in service of patient centricity.

WHAT ARE THE RAMIFICATIONS OF EXTREME HONESTY AFTER PATIENT HARM?
Case (Continued)

After the operating room fire, a focused case review is conducted. The performance data review uncovers the expected risk factors for fire, including high-flow oxygen, alcohol preparation solutions, and an increased bleeding risk. The antagonistic microculture in the operating room also surfaces, as do prior traumatic learning experiences affecting Nurse Corage, the obstetrics and gynecology nurse involved, and Dr Lerner, the anesthesia resident. The event review is limited, however, relying on most common way of fact finding: having all professionals involved in the event mustered together in a room. There, Dr Scalpelle's intimidating demeanor dampens the free exchange of information.

On an uncoordinated parallel track, the university's risk management office is asked to respond to the patient and family, who are increasingly expressing their frustration. They have been told nothing since Dr Scalpelle and Dr Propofal asked for permission to examine the patient's airway at time of the fire. Risk management, circumspect about the threat of litigation, reaches out to the patient and family. Resolved to share only "concrete" information related to the events of the operating room that led to the fire, the exchange is sterile—and offensive. The patient and family are reminded that they signed a consent form, which detailed an encyclopedic list of risks, including death.

Medical ethicists have long held that physicians have a duty to tell patients the truth about unplanned clinical outcomes. Wu and colleagues[8] traced the concept at least back to the American Medical Association's Principles of Medical Ethics published in 1957; however, at the time, most physicians interpreted the statement as a duty to report to a risk management committee, not the patient. The gulf between patients' expectations and actual practices widened over ensuing decades. Deferring communications to the risk management office spared health professionals from answering difficult questions, but it came at the price of sacrificing the caring relationship between the patient and the clinician. Patients felt abandoned, and the family—often privately guilty that they did not somehow do more to prevent the harm—developed a profound distrust of the organization and anyone associated with it.

Despite the ethical imperative to move beyond deny-and-defend practices, the idea of talking transparently with patients and families about harm was regarded with great skepticism. Although attitudes are changing, this skepticism remains strong today. Conventional wisdom held that financial catastrophe would result from unvarnished honesty. Prominent scholars estimated that only 2% of medical errors causing injury ever came to the attention of lawyers, leading them to surmise that American medicine could ill afford to unleash "a huge reservoir of potential claims" by being honest about mistakes that harmed patients. They predicted that widespread disclosure could threaten the very foundations of medicine, asserting, "That severe injuries are prevalent and that most of them never trigger litigation are epidemiologic facts that have long been evident. The affordability of the medical malpractice system rests on this fragile foundation, and routine disclosure threatens to shake it."[9,10]

Yet, some openly questioned the ethics and financial assumptions of deny-and-defend practices. Albert Wu has long championed physicians' ethical and professional obligations.[11] In 1999, Dr Steve Kraman and attorney Ginny Hamm published an article titled, "Risk Management: Extreme Honesty May Be the Best Policy,"[12] where they described an "extreme honesty" approach implemented at Lexington, Kentucky, Veteran's Administration (VA) Hospital. They landmark study revealed that financial catastrophe did not ensue when their "humanistic risk management policy" claims track record was compared with other similarly situated VA hospitals. The study had a major limitation, however—that claims against the VA hospital system are governed by the Federal Tort Claims Act, which requires patients to name only the US government and to take their case first before an administrative law judge. The authors acknowledged that private hospital systems would face barriers not present in a VA hospital.

HOW CAN BARRIERS TO TRANSPARENCY BE SURMOUNTED? ENTER THE MICHIGAN MODEL

In 2001, the University of Michigan also dared to question the usefulness of deny and defend and mapped out what has become known as the Michigan Model, a proactive and principled response to adverse patient outcomes (**Fig. 4**). The approach serves as the main template for today's communication and resolution program model. It differed from the Lexington VA's approach in that it was motivated not only by the sense of professional ethical obligations to harmed individual patients and families, but also by a stalwart conviction that deny and defend was damaging the clinical mission.

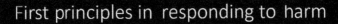

First principles in responding to harm

Honesty

Honesty is the transcendent core value that makes everything else possible. It is the north star that guides the path taken and in doing so elevates the clinical mission.

Transparency

Transparency refers to openness and accountability, shining a light on the truth around an adverse event. Transparency is only possible when extreme honesty pervades the organization.

Courage

Courage is the moral rectitude to overcome fear and to act with integrity. Courage overcomes counterproductive denial and defensiveness, which impede efforts to improve care.

Fig. 4. Tenets of communication and resolution programs.

By 2002, validated by early claims experience, the self-insured University of Michigan Health System freed itself from the need for (and considerable expense of) excess coverage. This transition allowed even greater autonomy in how the university elected to respond to patients who experienced unintended harm. With enthusiastic support from its clinical leadership, the institution proceeded to a radical transformation of the organization's claims management approach. The traditional reactive strategy of waiting for lawsuits to surface was replaced by a proactive and principled strategy to unfavorable patient care outcomes. The model leverages clinician insight into when avoidable deficiencies in care caused harm and adapts accordingly.

Whereas the deny-and-defend edifice asks, "Is this case defensible?" the Michigan Model asks, "Did the care at issue meet our clinical expectations?" The latter question is far more aligned with the medical mission. The 2 questions often yield very different outcomes. Defensibility depends on a host of factors, many entirely unrelated to care—the likeability of the parties, the availability of experts on either side, the quality of the attorneys, the magnitude of the calculable and incalculable damages, the statutes of limitations, state laws, civil procedure rules, and geography. Social attitudes may also influence the courtroom verdict. In his essay entitled, *Liars Don't Always Lose*, Jacob Stein observed: "The truth lawyers see is ... always a truth combined with something else. There is the taint related to bias and prejudice. There is the taint of deliberate falsehood." Physicians have traditionally enjoyed favorable bias, continuing to present day—especially in underserved geographies and buoyed by the "health care heroes" of the pandemic. Often, care that does not meet clinical expectations may be legally defensible, but defending it undermines efforts at professionalism, high reliability, patient safety, and patient centricity.

Thus, honesty became the founding principle of the Michigan Model and is the foundation of all authentic communication and resolution programs. Honesty drives the organizational response to the affected patients and families. Perhaps more important, this emphasis on honesty was a necessary predicate to the continual clinical improvement that protects future patients and health care professionals from the trauma of repeated patient harm. When lawyers, insurance professionals, and risk managers mold the organization's response to injured patients based on the question

"Is this case defensible?" they risk moral injury in the clinical staff if an honest clinical assessment fails to line up with the courtroom-driven response. In contrast, all of the elements of the Michigan Model intentionally align with clinical values.[1,2,13–17]

The nine elements of the Michigan Model are:

1. Capture all unintended clinical outcomes regardless of the perceived cause—delay in recognizing harm exposes others to the same risk.
2. Secure the clinical environment to ensure no other patient is harmed as the investigation proceeds.
3. Get to the bedside as soon as possible and engage the patient and family with compassion and without defensiveness. Clinical and risk management staff are selected for emotional intelligence and trained to always show empathy. They reassure the patient and family that the patient will not be abandoned, promising to share facts as quickly as they are known. Listening is critical not only to a sincere empathic response; patients often have important information not routinely gathered as part of most root cause analyses[18]—communication lines between risk management and those responsible for clinical improvement are purposefully streamlined.
4. Engage the health care professionals involved with compassion and purpose to ensure they are fully supported emotionally as they cope with the unplanned clinical outcome and to ensure that they are safe for duty.
5. Normalize honesty with a rigorous investigation and assessment reaching clinical conclusions as to the reasonableness of care, cause, and extent of injury.
6. Transparently share facts and conclusions with caregivers and patients; then share these facts widely within the organization as warranted. "Disclosure" is a process, rarely a single conversation and rarely attempted in the heat of the moment. It is always disciplined, thoughtful, and honest.
7. Follow through completely and consistently, implementing patient safety improvements, peer review, and fiscal resolution with the patient, if warranted. Monitor the response to clinical changes for effectiveness and durability.
8. Leverage lessons learned to enhance patient safety, breaking down traditional divisions between patient safety and quality offices and the risk management or legal offices.
9. Measure metrics that advance the clinical mission, evaluating patient safety improvements, tracking patient and clinical staff satisfaction, and measuring the true financial cost of lapses in quality or safety.

Some of the key operational differences between the model and "deny-and-defend" include the following.

- *Responsiveness*: The organization does not wait for a claim, nor for someone to ask for compensation; instead, it proactively responds to any unanticipated clinical outcome.
- *Patient-centric:* Health professionals maintain the relationship with the patient and family after an adverse clinical outcome, attending to needs regardless of findings of peer review
- *Clinical standard:* Substandard clinical care is not blindly defended. Also, unplanned clinical outcomes that did not result from inappropriate care are not considered for compensation.
- *Patient safety focus:* Peer review and clinical improvements to protect against future harm is are not delayed or sidetracked by litigation concerns around a possible courtroom defense.

- *Known cost of failures:* Organizations can place a reliable cost on failures of care, encouraging capital decisions that prioritize safety and quality.

Compared with traditional litigation responses to patient harm, every element of communication and resolution programs promotes the clinical mission for individual health care professionals and organizations alike. Although not the primary intention of the programs, the model has also delivered claims costs savings, which can support rapidly implemented clinical care improvements.[19] The model has served the University of Michigan's health system and clinical staff well for nearly 2 decades and has been adopted by several health care organizations around the country.[20] There are now hundreds of hospitals with communication and resolution programs in place, demonstrating varying degrees of rigor in implementation.

PRACTICAL STEPS FOR TALKING TO PATIENTS WITH EMPATHY AND TRUST

Sharing an unexpected patient safety event is stressful for a patient's loved ones. Guidance on how to approach the initial harm conversation with patients and family is given in **Fig. 5**. It is best to find a location that is quiet, minimizes distractions, and allows everyone a place to sit. Body language should convey openness, making eye contact, leaning forward attentively, and avoiding crossed arms. After the family is informed of the patient's status, the known facts of the adverse event are shared. As in a motor vehicle accident, speculating on unknowns or fault is usually counterproductive; instead, convey next steps. The family should be invited to share their concerns, and the clinician should not become defensive. Mirroring helps to ensure that the family is being heard, and listening with empathy builds trust and avoids misunderstanding. There are significant differences in how patients and physicians rate the quality of harm conversations, with physicians often having a significantly more optimistic view than their patients (**Fig. 6**). The quality of these conversations can be enhanced with empathy.

Empathy includes attunement, which involves emotional and somatic resonance—tuning into the experience of another—along with the cognitive dimension of perspective taking. It also requires humility—holding lightly to what we think we know and

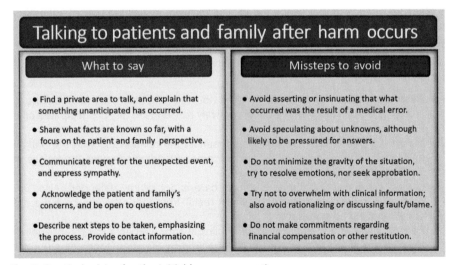

Fig. 5. Practical advice for the initial harm conversation.

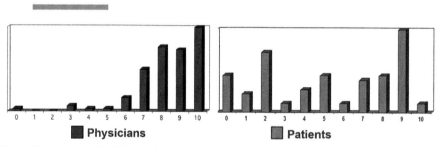

Fig. 6. Patient and physician rating of quality of harm conversation. Ratings of quality of harm conversation on a scale of 0 (extremely low quality) to 10 (extremely high quality). (Unpublished data, Courtesy of Thomas H. Gallagher, MD, University of Washington.)

allowing for the discovery of something new. The elements are coupled with curiosity and openness. The nonverbal awareness of where the other person is emotionally does not always involve strong shared feeling, but this empathy facilitates trust and may allow for involuntary matching of nonverbal style, such as vocal tones. Empathy can be cultivated through interest, curiosity, and caring about others. When trying to grasp what the family is experiencing, we may find ourselves resonating with them, which is a backdrop to attunement. The cognitive aspect of clinical empathy involves discerning emotional states and labeling them cand also improve the quality of the interaction. Empathy helps to build trust, decreases anxiety, and affords an experiential approach to comprehending emotional states.[21]

Emotional intelligence—which refers to the capacity to recognize and manage one's own feelings and to recognize and respond to the feeling of others—also has an important role in navigating harm conversations. It can help us control our own reactions and be receptive to those of others. Training in emotional intelligence allows for creation of high-functioning teams with high empathy. Daniel Goleman's 4 domains of emotional intelligence include self-awareness (emotional self-awareness, self-assessment, and self-confidence), social awareness (empathy, organizational awareness, and service), self-regulation (emotional self-control, transparency, adaptability, achievement, initiative, and optimism), and relationship management (influence, leadership, navigating conflict, teamwork, and collaboration).[22]

Patients and family members need clarity about how the process will unfold. The family should be kept informed of progress in understanding what happened and assured as to what measures are being taken avoid future injury to other patients. They should also be given an opportunity to be part of the solution. A follow-up meeting should be arranged to discuss progress, and the family is provided contact information so that they can call with questions or concerns. The response to harm with the communication and resolution program loosely corresponds with the components of a plan–do–study–act cycle (**Fig. 7**).

HOW WOULD A COMMUNICATION AND RESOLUTION PROGRAM CHANGE THE RESPONSE TO THE SURGICAL FIRE?

Communication and response programs are based on honesty and afford a variety of benefits over traditional approaches to unexpected clinical outcomes (**Fig. 8**). Reporting also plays a vital role—both in detecting near misses and responding to harm; if Dr Propofal had realized the toxic impact of Dr Scalpelle's recurring disrespectful behaviors, it would trigger his own duty to protect others. With the benefit of reporting, Dr Scalpelle

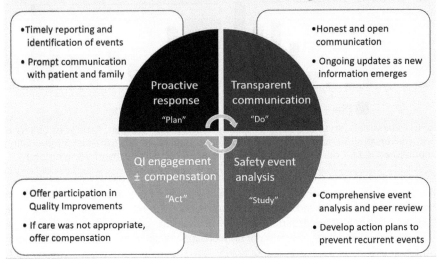

Fig. 7. Plan–do–study–act (PDSA) cycle conceptualization of response to adverse events. QI, quality improvement.

would likely have been called out earlier in his career, giving him a chance to reflect, get help, and modify his behavior before a fire ever occurred. After a fire does occur, the communication and resolution program makes future fires far less likely.

With a communication and resolution program, the fire would be reported immediately to the operating room leadership, to the patient safety office, and to clinical leaders. The program's performance profile would track the environment, key steps (reporting, communication, event analysis, and resolution), response to safety events, and outcomes (**Fig. 9**). Immediate steps would be taken to raise awareness and ensure that no other patients would be similarly harmed while the incident was being further studied. Alcohol-based preparation solutions might be removed from the area, or other interim steps necessary to mitigate similar risks would be taken. A member of the risk management team would meet the family while their loved one was still in the

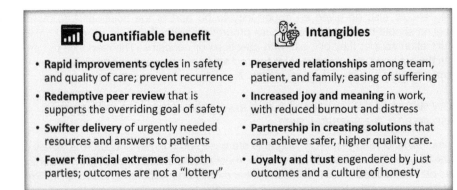

Fig. 8. Benefits conferred by communication and resolution programs.

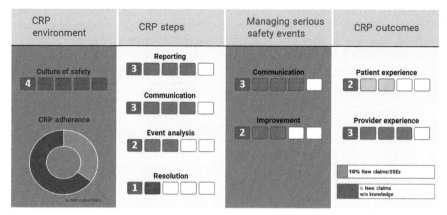

Fig. 9. Communication and resolution program (CRP) program profile. This dashboard allows an institution to track how successful its implementation efforts are from environment, to key steps, to quality improvement procedures and outcomes. (*From* Ariadne Labs and the University of Washington.)

operating room or in the recovery unit, communicating with empathy, listening carefully, and offering a solid promise to keep them informed.

Few incidents are completely understood immediately, and more harm can be done with an undisciplined and false explanation than with one delayed long enough to know the difference between fact and conjecture—rarely does the risk management consultant try to explain what happened in the heat of the moment. The risk manager might respond to the family's insistence on answers by explaining, "I understand your questions—we share them ourselves—and we will move as quickly as possible to get to the bottom of it, but it would be disrespectful to you and all concerned for me to speculate right now. Let's focus on your loved one's needs and I promise that as we nail down the details, we will share them with you. In the meantime, we are taking positive steps to protect other patients and staff."

From that point forward, the patient's needs, the family's needs, and the caregivers' needs would be foremost in the assigned risk manager's mind, and lines of communication with the patient and family would be established. Managing information expectations is critical. The patient and family would also be advised that the organization would not treat them any differently if they felt the need to have a lawyer and offered a list of top malpractice plaintiff's lawyers with a history of working constructively with the organization.

As soon as possible, the clinical staff involved would also be engaged and debriefed. Their own trauma would be addressed. Operating room fires are dramatic events and often clinical staff worry for their own safety. The connection between the emotional and physical health of caregivers and the quality and safety of the care they deliver is inarguable. The staff should be treated with empathy, care, and attention to their suitability for service. Organizations that operate communication and resolution programs are encouraged to have resources at the ready, including prearranged avenues to relieve any health care professionals from service if felt not to be safe; this measure is for their own safety and that of coworkers and patients.

After the initial discussion with the family, debriefing the clinical staff, and taking steps to minimize the risk of another fire, an investigation is conducted immediately, and the facts are assessed. Clinical leaders are notified and asked to weigh in on the care to build a sense of shared ownership of the clinical events and necessary measures. Where appropriate, outside experts may be sought to get to the bottom of what happened clinically as quickly as possible. The experts are not to develop a defense, but rather to either guard against defensive bias in the assessment or to obtain expertise. If harm was determined to have arisen from care that was felt to be unreasonable or failed to meet expectations, discussions around compensation would follow.

MODERN COMMUNICATION AND RESOLUTION PROGRAMS

The Agency for Healthcare Research and Quality launched a $23 million Patient Safety and Medical Liability grant initiative to accelerate the implementation of communication and resolution programs. In 2016, the agency unveiled the CANDOR toolkit, a roadmap for creating communication and resolution programs; a schematic of the approach is shown in **Fig. 10**.[23] Widespread adoption of the model had previously been slow and with inconsistent implementation. With the recent acceleration in adoption, many institutions have launched programs, although many have focused primarily on the claims management component of the model. Limited implementations overlook the considerable benefits of aligning the response to patient[14,24–27] harm, with the larger clinical mission of delivering safe, high-quality care.[28]

In recent years, there have been notable successes with signal initiatives.[24,29,30] For example, a remarkably successful undertaking, The Massachusetts Alliance for Communication and Resolution following Medical Injury (MACRMI) grew out of the original Agency for Healthcare Research and Quality initiatives (https://www.macrmi.info/). MACRMI continues to prove the concept. Starting with only 6 hospitals, it now has more than 20 members organizations and continues to grow. MACRMI

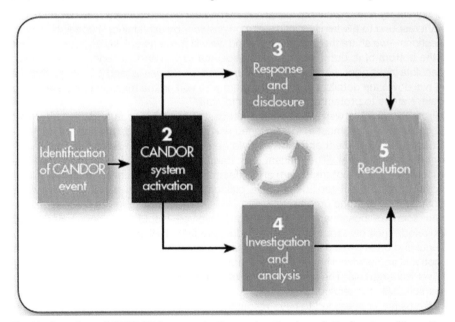

Fig. 10. Overview of CANDOR (communication and optimal resolution) system. (*From* "Implementation Guide for the CANDOR Process." Communication and Optimal Resolution (CANDOR). (Content last reviewed February 2017). Agency for Healthcare Research and Quality; Rockville, MD. https://www.ahrq.gov/patient-safety/capacity/candor/impguide.html.)

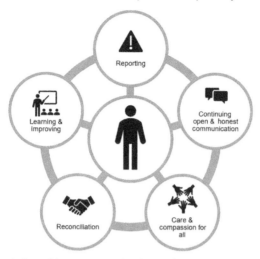

Fig. 11. Pictorial depiction of how communication and resolutions foster patient centricity. (Reproduced with permission, courtesy of Collaborative for Accountability and Improvement, Patient and Family Advocate Committee, University of Washington, Copyright 2020.)

generously shares its experience and processes. An important observation regarding all communication and resolution programs is that the term "resolution" refers to instating improvement measures and compensating for harm when the care was not acceptable; it should in no way be taken to mean that closure or resolution for the family has been achieved, for patients or their loved ones will often carry the weight of harm for a lifetime.

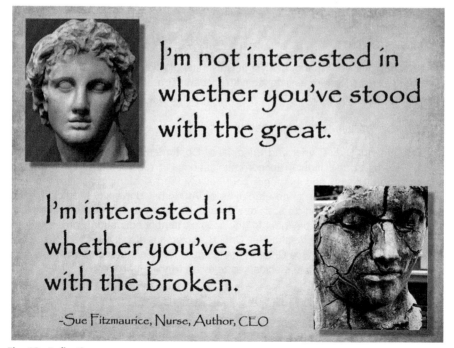

Fig. 12. Reflection.

Another national resource is The Collaborative for Accountability and Improvement (CAI). It serves as a clearing house for best practices, including patient and family resources (**Fig. 11**). The contribution of CAI is in bringing together stakeholders and resources to disseminate knowledge and support implementation. In the past, attorneys—especially health care organizations' defense lawyers and defense trial lawyers—had greeted this model with skepticism and even hostility. CAI has now formed the CRP Attorney Alliance, a new group composed of lawyers on all sides of the patient injury and medical malpractice process. Lawyers from the defense trial bar, general counsel, health care lawyers, plaintiff's trial lawyers, and academic law professors have joined this fledgling group.

SUMMARY

When a patient is harmed, the traditional response has been defensiveness and stonewalling, which erodes trust. This reflexive response, rooted in denial, lacks empathy and compassion; it deepens emotional suffering for the patient, family members, and health care professionals. It also undermines efforts to improve care and prevent future harm. As an alternative to the deny-and-defend paradigm, communication and resolution programs provide a principled and comprehensive approach for responding to unintended patient harm, emphasizing honesty and transparency across the care continuum. These programs are designed to reinforce the patient–clinician relationship, address the needs of patients harmed during their care, and promote continual improvement. It keeps clinicians at the side of patients and families in the aftermath of harm (**Fig. 12**). To succeed, the programs must be prioritized by the organization, aligned with the clinical mission, and have buy-in from institutional leaders. The approach's emphasis on empathic communication supports the well-being of health care professionals. In Part 3 of this series, the vignette continues to unfold, illuminating the third pillar, wellness, and resilience.

ACKNOWLEDGMENTS

The authors thank Yan Zhang, analyst in University of Michigan Office of Patient Relations and Clinical Risk for assistance with preparing data on the Michigan Model for analysis and inclusion in this article.

CONFLICT OF INTEREST AND DISCLOSURE

R.C. Boothman, JD, is Owner and Principal of Boothman Consulting, which assists health systems in transitioning to communication and resolutions programs, conducting programmatic and personal peer review, and designing peer review approaches. Dr G.B. Hickson is an employee of Vanderbilt University Medical Center and is a member of Medtronic's speakers bureau. He receives royalties from Cognitive Institute; and has received payment for the development of educational presentations from numerous health care institutions. Dr G.B. Hickson is also a member of the USC Health System Board and Vice Chair of the Institute for Healthcare Improvement (IHI) Board. No other authors have disclosures relevant to this publication.

REFERENCES

1. Boothman RC, Blackwell AC, Campbell DA Jr, et al. A better approach to medical malpractice claims? The University of Michigan experience. J Health Life Sci Law 2009;2(2):125–59.

2. Boothman RC, Imhoff SJ, Campbell DA Jr. Nurturing a culture of patient safety and achieving lower malpractice risk through disclosure: lessons learned and future directions. Front Health Serv Manage 2012;28(3):13–28.

3. Brenner MJ, Chang CWD, Boss EF, et al. Patient safety/quality improvement primer, part I: what PS/QI means to your otolaryngology practice. Otolaryngol Head Neck Surg 2018;159(1):3–10.

4. Brenner MJ. A piece of my mind. Collateral damage. JAMA 2009;301(16): 1637–8.

5. Hickson GB, Clayton EW, Githens PB, et al. Factors that prompted families to file medical malpractice claims following perinatal injuries. JAMA 1992;267(10): 1359–63.

6. Vincent C, Young M, Phillips A. Why do people sue doctors? A study of patients and relatives taking legal action. Lancet 1994;343(8913):1609–13.

7. Console RP. Bad bedside manner or medical malpractice? Natl L Rev 2021;11(2).

8. Wu AW, Cavanaugh TA, McPhee SJ, et al. To tell the truth: ethical and practical issues in disclosing medical mistakes to patients. J Gen Intern Med 1997; 12(12):770–5.

9. Studdert DM, Mello MM, Gawande AA, et al. Claims, errors, and compensation payments in medical malpractice litigation. N Engl J Med 2006;354(19):2024–33.

10. Studdert DM, Mello MM, Gawande AA, et al. Disclosure of medical injury to patients: an improbable risk management strategy. Health Aff (Millwood) 2007; 26(1):215–26.

11. Wu AW, Boyle DJ, Wallace G, et al. Disclosure of adverse events in the United States and Canada: an update, and a proposed framework for improvement. J Public Health Res 2013;2(3):e32.

12. Kraman SS, Hamm G. Risk management: extreme honesty may be the best policy. Ann Intern Med 1999;131(12):963–7.

13. Biermann JS, Boothman R. There is another approach to medical malpractice disputes. J Oncol Pract 2006;2(4):148.

14. Boothman R, Gallagher T, Woodward A. Health systems turn to communication and resolution programs to identify errors. ED Manag 2017;29(6):S1–4.

15. Boothman R, Hoyler MM. The University of Michigan's early disclosure and offer program. Bull Am Coll Surg 2013;98(3):21–5.

16. Boothman RC, Blackwell AC. Integrating risk management activities into a patient safety program. Clin Obstet Gynecol 2010;53(3):576–85.

17. Taheri PA, Butz DA, Anderson S, et al. Medical liability-the crisis, the reality, and the data: the University of Michigan story. J Am Coll Surg 2006;203(3):290–6.

18. Balakrishnan K, Brenner MJ, Gosbee JW, et al. Patient safety/quality improvement primer, part II: prevention of harm through root cause analysis and action (RCA(2)). Otolaryngol Head Neck Surg 2019;161(6):911–21.

19. Kachalia A, Kaufman SR, Boothman R, et al. Liability claims and costs before and after implementation of a medical error disclosure program. Ann Intern Med 2010;153(4):213–21.

20. Sage WM, Boothman RC, Gallagher TH. Another medical malpractice crisis? Try something different. JAMA 2020;324(14):1395–6.

21. Halpern J. What is clinical empathy? J Gen Intern Med 2003;18(8):670–4.

22. Goleman D. Working with emotional intelligence. New York: Bantam Books; 1998.

23. Boothman RC. CANDOR: the antidote to deny and defend? Health Serv Res 2016;51(Suppl 3):2487–90.

24. Gallagher TH, Boothman RC, Schweitzer L, et al. Making communication and resolution programmes mission critical in healthcare organisations. BMJ Qual Saf 2020;29(11):875–8.
25. Gallagher TH, Mello MM, Sage WM, et al. Can communication-and-resolution programs achieve their potential? five key questions. Health Aff (Millwood) 2018;37(11):1845–52.
26. Mello MM, Armstrong SJ, Greenberg Y, et al. Challenges of implementing a communication-and-resolution program where multiple organizations must cooperate. Health Serv Res 2016;51(Suppl 3):2550–68.
27. Sage WM, Gallagher TH, Armstrong S, et al. How policy makers can smooth the way for communication-and- resolution programs. Health Aff (Millwood) 2014; 33(1):11–9.
28. Bell SK, Smulowitz PB, Woodward AC, et al. Disclosure, apology, and offer programs: stakeholders' views of barriers to and strategies for broad implementation. Milbank Q 2012;90(4):682–705.
29. Gallagher TH, Boothman RC, Schweitzer L, et al. Key marketing message for communication and resolution programmes: the authors reply. BMJ Qual Saf 2020;29(9):779.
30. Mello MM, Boothman RC, McDonald T, et al. Communication-and-resolution programs: the challenges and lessons learned from six early adopters. Health Aff (Millwood) 2014;33(1):20–9.

Honesty and Transparency, Indispensable to the Clinical Mission—Part III

How Leaders Can Prevent Burnout, Foster Wellness and Recovery, and Instill Resilience

Michael J. Brenner, MD[a,b,]*, Gerald B. Hickson, MD[c,d],
Richard C. Boothman, JD[c,e,f], Cynda Hylton Rushton, PhD, RN[g,h,i],
Carol R. Bradford, MD, MS[j,k]

KEYWORDS

- Burnout • Wellness • Well-being • Resilience • Ethics • Moral resilience
- Depersonalization • Emotional exhaustion

Continued

Disclosures/Conflict of Interest: Dr Hickson is an employee of Vanderbilt University Medical Center and is a member of Medtronic's speakers bureau. He receives royalties from Cognitive Institute and has received payment for the development of educational presentations from numerous health care institutions. Dr Hickson is also a member of the USC Health System Board and Vice Chair of the Institute for Healthcare Improvement (IHI) Board.
Professor Cynda Hylton Rushton is the Editor of the book <u>Moral Resilience: Transforming Moral Suffering in Healthcare</u> (2018) and receives royalties for this publication.
Dr Bradford has been a visiting professor speaking about well-being/wellness at Henry Ford and University of Kansas Otolaryngology departments and received an honorarium for these engagements.
[a] Associate Professor, Department of Otolaryngology – Head & Neck Surgery, University of Michigan Medical School, 1500 East Medical Center Drive, 1903 Taubman Center, SPC 5312, Ann Arbor, MI 48104, USA; [b] GTC Quality Improvement Collaborative, Durham, NC, USA; [c] Center for Patient and Professional Advocacy, Vanderbilt University Medical Center, Nashville, TN, USA; [d] Center for Quality, Safety and Risk Prevention, Vanderbilt University Medical Center, Nashville, TN, USA; [e] Boothman Consulting Group, LLC, Ann Arbor, MI, USA; [f] Department of Surgery, University of Michigan Medical School, Ann Arbor, MI, USA; [g] Johns Hopkins University School of Nursing, Baltimore, MD, USA; [h] Department of Pediatrics, Johns Hopkins University School of Medicine, Baltimore, MD, USA; [i] Berman Institute of Bioethics, Johns Hopkins University School of Medicine, Baltimore, MD, USA; [j] The College of Medicine and James Cancer Hospital and Solove Research Institute; [k] Department of Otolaryngology-Head and Neck Surgery, The Ohio State University Wexner Medical Center, Columbus, OH, USA
* Corresponding author. Department of Otolaryngology-Head & Neck Surgery, University of Michigan School of Medicine, 1500 East Medical Center Drive SPC 5312, 1904 Taubman Center, Ann Arbor, MI 48109-5312.
E-mail address: mbren@med.umich.edu

Continued

KEY POINTS

- Burnout syndrome, comprising emotional exhaustion, depersonalization, and diminished sense of personal accomplishment, can be greatly magnified in the wake of a patient safety event.
- Burnout harms patients and threatens health care professionals; burnout is strongly associated with surgeon self-reported errors, and deleterious effects may be even more pervasive among nurses.
- Moral distress is an emotional state that arises when a person feels compelled to take actions that diverge from what is thought to be ethically correct; persons may feel powerless, anxious, and depressed.
- Moral resilience is the ability of an individual to preserve or restore integrity in response to moral adversity; moral courage refers to the strength to speak up despite the fear of repercussions.
- Leaders have a critical role in restoring joy in work and fostering workplace resilience, through mitigating drivers of burnout, modeling wellness, and fostering relational integrity.

When we learn how to become resilient, we learn how to embrace the beautifully broad spectrum of the human experience.

-Jaeda DeWalt, artist and writer

INTRODUCTION

Burnout and moral injury have come to forefront of health care, accounting for surges in staff turnover, spiraling rates of mental illness, and critical shortages of frontline professionals. At the sharp end of care—where harm can arise from a slip of a scalpel, loss of an airway, or injection from a mislabeled syringe—our proximity to adverse events is palpable. Seemingly lesser slips—failure to wash our hands, to put on a mask, or to respond to a page—can also harm patients and degrade care. Any such experience can sow doubt, erode trust, and wound morale of health care professionals, who routinely contend with long work hours, high levels of stress, and intense emotional and physical strain. From both a humanitarian and sustainability perspective, leaders must therefore be purposeful in championing wellness and resilience.

This final component of the 3-part series explores how ensuring the well-being of health care professionals advances the clinical mission (**Fig. 1**). Building on insights from the preceding 2 sections, *Part 3* examines the drivers of burnout and the invisible wound of moral injury. It discusses these 2 phenomena in detail—how they differ and what can be done to alleviate them. The leadership strategies presented encompass not only how leaders can address root causes of suffering but also how to instill resilience through shared human experience, mutual respect, and relational integrity. Visionary leaders champion psychological safety, create the learning systems, and foster collective resilience. A hypothetical clinical vignette initiated within the prior 2 parts continues in this final part, interspersing a narrative foundation for discussing best practices for restoring joy, meaning, and purpose in work.

CASE PRESENTATION

*In **Parts 1 and 2**, Dr Scalpelle (attending surgeon) engaged in uncivil interactions with other members of the surgical team, flouting safety practices and risking harm. When a surgical fire ensues, the patient suffers burns, and the patient, family, and healthcare*

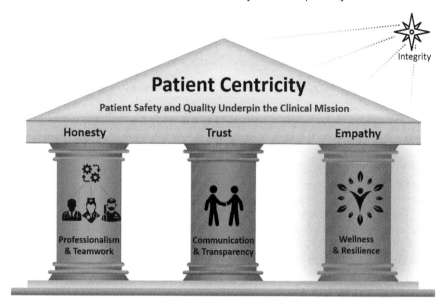

Fig. 1. Values-driven framework for improving honesty and transparency around adverse events. The core values of honesty, trust, and empathy are the basis for delivering safe, high-quality care. *Professionalism and Teamwork (Part 1)* introduced tiered interventions that promote professional accountability. *Communication and Transparency (Part 2)* offered a principled approach for responding to patient harm. *Wellness and Resilience (Part 3)* is the culmination of the preceding parts, initially exploring drivers of burnout and moral injury and then presenting leadership solutions to restore joy in work and integrity.

*team all suffer trauma. **Part 3** travels the rocky road to recovery as the team members progress from burnout and moral adversity to resilience.*

Following discussion of the operating room fire at Morbidity and Mortality conference, Dr Scalpelle walls himself off, avoiding contact with the patient and with family—who still have questions. The residents and staff observe that Dr Scalpelle is abrupt with them, and nurses have requested not to be assigned to Dr Scalpelle's room, which is causing disruptions in team dynamics and staffing. A colleague takes Dr Scalpelle for a cup of coffee to review concerns reported anonymously. Dr Scalpelle is indignant. "There's *nothing* wrong!" he barks, exiting abruptly, his coffee left on the table.

Consider a few opening questions:

- What are the consequences of disruptive or avoidant behavior on teamwork and safety?
- When is it time to escalate the response, given the disturbances rippling through the system?
- Are Dr Scalpelle's colleagues and leadership even aware of resources that might help?

Others on the team are also affected. Dr Lerner, the anesthesia resident who was compelled to dial up the oxygen just before the operating room fire, has been listless and distracted; he is having difficulty focusing and recently made a medication dosing error. When asked about the error, he admits to feeling disconnected from his work and his patients. Dr Propofol, the attending anesthesiologist, went on sabbatical; she has been unreachable. Dr Resedent, the surgical resident, admits she has experienced intrusive thoughts, worrying about a lawsuit.

A few follow-up questions:

- What is the significance of the differing reactions of the physician members of the team?
- How should Dr Lerner's loss of engagement with patients and his training be addressed?
- As the effects of the operating room fire spread out across team members, what can be done?

The Hidden Epidemic of Burnout in Health Professionals

Clinicians—across all disciplines and care settings—are experiencing alarming rates of burnout, which is characterized by work exhaustion and interpersonal disengagement.[1] Before the pandemic, 35% to 54% of nurses and physicians and 45% to 60% of medical students and residents reported experiencing substantial symptoms of burnout.[2] In the COVID-19 pandemic era, burnout has intensified.[3] The deleterious effects of burnout on clinicians and learners include increased risk for occupational injury, stunted professional development, alcohol or drug dependency, and mental illness. Nurses may have increased risk of burnout because of their responsibility for most of the moment-to-moment care of patients.

Burnout also has dire effects on the financial health of organizations, potentially interfering with operations or ability to adequately fund safety or quality initiatives.[4–6] Physicians with work exhaustion and disengagement are more likely to reduce their work load,[7] leave their current job or go on sabbatical,[8,9] or depart from patient care altogether (**Fig. 2**).[7] Similar findings, in some instances even more pronounced, are evident across the nursing profession.[3,10–12] Clinician burnout is associated with lower patient satisfaction, reduced quality and safety of care, and increased risk of suicide.[13–18] In addition, patient complaints are more likely in clinicians with burnout, and clinicians who accrue more complaints may experience higher rates of surgical complications and malpractice claims.[19–21]

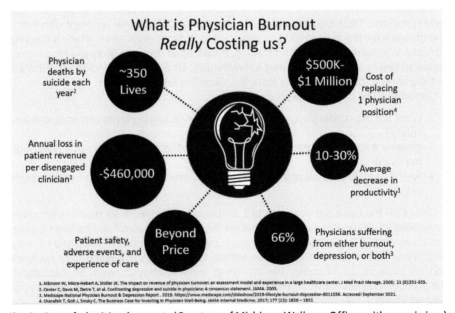

Fig. 2. Cost of physician burnout. (*Courtesy of* Michigan Wellness Office; with permission.)

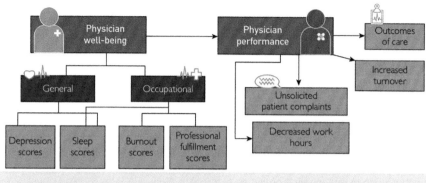

Proposed Relationship among Physician Wellness, Performance and Outcomes of Care

Fig. 3. The link between clinician well-being and performance. (*From* Welle, et. al., Association of Occupational Distress and Sleep-Related Impairment in Physicians With Unsolicited Patient Complaints, Mayo Clinic Proceedings, Volume 95, Issue 4, 2020, Pages 719-726, ISSN 0025-6196, https://doi.org/10.1016/j.mayocp.2019.09.025. (https://www.sciencedirect.com/science/article/pii/S0025619619308730.)

Prior studies have also demonstrated a strong relationship between clinician burnout, self-reported medical errors, and patient care outcomes.[15,22,23] Each point increase in a surgeon's self-reported emotional exhaustion score corresponds to a 5-point increase in errors—a negative association that doubles for depersonalization scores.[18] Reduced safety and quality of care, reduced patient satisfaction, and mental

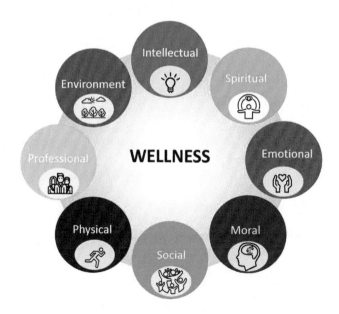

Fig. 4. Wellness domains.

and physical fatigue all occur with burnout.[18] There is also a link between risk of burnout and volume of clinical care; the more heavily clinical a health professionals' role, the greater the severity of burnout typically observed—especially if the system is not committed to pursuing effective teams.[3] A model explaining the link between physician wellness and performance is shown in **Fig. 3**.

How Can Leaders Promote Wellness and Resilience?

Leaders need to invest in the occupation-specific well-being of health care professionals, which involves implementing strategies to promote wellness and resilience. Wellness is the pursuit of activities that promote personal integrity and wholeness, and its domains are depicted in **Fig. 4**. Resilience relates to the ability to resolve conflict and recover from emotional or physical injury. It involves rediscovering joy in work and engaging in replenishing activities external to the workplace such as physical exercise, art, prayer, or family. Resilience also has an internal aspect that involves mitigating traumatic experiences, cherishing the value of life despite inevitable hardships, and nourishing a sense of hope, meaning, and purpose. An enhanced capacity to meet challenges can protect against both burnout and moral adversity, so leaders who model wellness can inspire health in their organizations.

Effective leaders must also address negative influences—including disruptive individuals whose unprofessional behavior can have far-reaching effects. The triad of people, organization, and systems summarize the necessary infrastructure to promote professional accountability (discussed in Part 1). It needs to be easy for team members to do the right thing, whether by reporting professional concerns or by abiding by professional standards themselves. The importance of teamwork for patient care and clinician wellness cannot be overstated. *To Err is Human*, which ushered in the modern patient safety era, emphasized building safer systems,[24] which had the unanticipated consequence of deemphasizing the vital role of professional accountability. In many cases, a recalibration is needed to ensure that there is a shared commitment by all professionals to create a safe environment.[25]

The operating room fire described in the case illustrates why professional accountability and safe systems are both needed. A system-oriented approach alone would

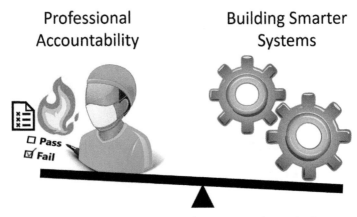

Fig. 5. Balancing individual responsibility and systems: underemphasis on professional accountability may overlook key safety considerations. (*Adapted from* Hickson, G.B. et al. Chapter 1: Balancing Systems and Individual Accountability in a Safety Culture. In: Front Office to Front Line: Essential Issues for Healthcare Leaders 2nd ed. Ed. Steven Berman. 2012. The Joint Commission International, A division of Joint Commission Resources, Inc.; with permission)

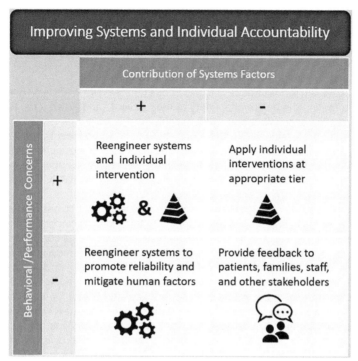

Fig. 6. Event analysis grid considering systems factors and individual factors. (*Adapted from* Hickson, G.B. et al. Chapter 1: Balancing Systems and Individual Accountability in a Safety Culture. In: Front Office to Front Line: Essential Issues for Healthcare Leaders 2nd ed. Ed. Steven Berman. 2012. The Joint Commission International, A division of Joint Commission Resources, Inc.; with permission.)

not detect the microculture that led to the surgical fire and all that followed. The prevailing underemphasis on personal accountability in many organizations is depicted in **Fig. 5**. Event analyses must therefore independently assess for behavioral/professional concerns *and* system failures, as depicted in **Fig. 6**. This approach helps ensure that preventable harm does not recur. In contrast, focusing solely on systems-based solutions overlooks well-being as requiring teamwork and systems. Clinician well-being supports a high-functioning care team, positive patient-clinician relationships, and an engaged workforce.

Robust approaches to ensuring personal accountability are particularly important for addressing events that require investigation, including physical contact, sexual boundary violation, or discrimination assertions. A huddle brings together stakeholders that include medical leaders, legal professionals, human resources, and nursing professionals. The huddle is designed to ensure a reliable, coordinated approach to address the problem and ensure safety for all involved parties. Those involved are generally senior leaders—those who have a right to know and who command the necessary people and systems. In an organization that espouses core values of honesty, trust, and empathy, the incidence of such events is rare, detection occurs early, and the culture reinforces resilience.

What Resources Do Health Care Professionals Require?

Leadership has a responsibility to develop and maintain an updated a list of well-being resources and sites for referral, also available from state boards and hospital associations. Small practice groups may argue that they cannot afford these resources, but this investment is critical to the success of the clinical mission. The faulty conclusion—that these provisions are too expensive—overlooks not only the moral duty to provide such resources but also the high monetary cost of losing professionals and managing complications, including preventable infections.[20,26,27]

The surgical team requires access to resources for their own well-being and to avoid negatively affecting the health and safety of their patients and coworkers. Resources should be readily accessible and customizable to the individual needs and preferences of health professionals. Furthermore, there need to be incentives to use these resources, and potential disincentives must be removed. For example, confidentiality is critical when accessing mental health services. Professionals also require time to devote to these activities within their workday, creating flexibility for using these resources.

Leadership engagement with front-line health care workers also has the potential to enhance the wellness and resilience within an organization. This engagement may be accomplished through town halls or using the Wellness Office as an organizing hub for departmental representatives who provide bidirectional input. A related approach is to empower clinical leaders in problem solving. By inviting the ideas and perspectives of clinical leaders at the departmental level, senior administrative leadership can improve the probability that solutions will be seen as practical and useful for front-line professionals. Having wellness champions across departments who meet regularly can foster a sense of community and lead to new well-being initiatives, including grant funding opportunities, seminars, and/or grand rounds to raise awareness, discuss best practices, and present case studies.

Last, a servant leadership philosophy and modeling wellness can benefit organizations. Servant leaders possess humility, courage, and service orientation. Intellectual curiosity is also a critically important attribute, as it allows leaders to learn, listen, and hear the voices of the people who they serve. Modeling wellness can be achieved by engaging in activities that support a healthy lifestyle and making these behaviors visible to members of the organization. In addition, leaders should embrace the concept of relational integrity, which is about acknowledging the interconnectedness of everyone's integrity, with the goal of creating environments where everyone is included and no one's integrity is diminished. The Institute for Healthcare Improvement Triple Aim describes how population health, experience of care, and attention to cost can guide health care, but more recently equity and team wellness or joy in work have been recognized as the missing piece in health care (**Fig. 7**).

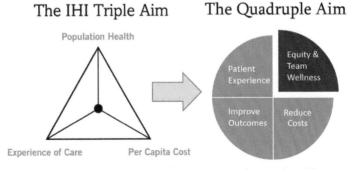

Fig. 7. Evolution from triple aim to quadruple aim adds professional well-being. The IHI Triple Aim framework was developed by the Institute for Healthcare Improvement in Boston, Massachusetts (http://www.ihi.org)

What Organizational Strategies to Burnout Are Available?

Drivers of baseline burnout at the organizational level are often linked to inefficient work processes, clerical burdens, and excessive workloads. Therefore, reengineering workflow can be beneficial in alleviating "work after work." Clinicians may feel that they are being reduced from front-line health care professionals to front-line data entry clerks, as they go about the business of managing overflowing in-baskets, entering orders, and reconciling medication. Identifying opportunities for incorporating scribes, advanced practice providers, patient portals, or voice recognition software may all reduce this burden.

In addition, adding flexibility, for example, allowing clinicians to conduct virtual visits from home, may alleviate conflicts between home and work duties. Baseline productivity pressures and stressors at home may also contribute—compounded in the colleague with a mental or physical health disorder, whose abilities are affected, generating fear and anger. Given the complexity of addressing burnout, it can be difficult to know what is working for individuals and clinicians collectively; therefore, leaders also require support in assessing progress of interventions.

Finally, leadership training on burnout should incorporate a variety of approaches, such as structured didactics, simulation/role playing, case-based learning, 360-degree feedback assessments, and one-on-one coaching. Leaders need partners and executive coaches to assess their progress in improving wellness, fostering health, and aiding recovery for clinicians. Cultivating soft skills can help ensure that leaders have the practical tools and conceptual framework to address these needs.

There are many additional approaches that leaders may promote as well. Examples include mindfulness huddles, gratitude journaling, biofeedback programs, compassion skills training, psychological safety training, reflective pauses, and well-being apps that allow for individual autonomy and flexibility in setting their own pace and routine. More relevant to the moral dimension of care are Schwartz huddles and postcode blue pause programs. Schwartz huddles are structured forums where staff, clinical and nonclinical, discuss the emotional and social aspects of working in health care. Postcode pause addresses the psychological and spiritual needs of code/trauma responders.[28,29] The next section delves more into the moral aspect of professional wellness.

CLINICAL CASE (CONTINUED)

Nurse Corage is asked by the chief of staff about the airway fire, and she describes the disrespectful interactions, neglected checklist, and other lapses of professional behavior. She is concerned that the family received only half of the story and is not being told what really happened in the operating room. She wonders whether the fire might have been prevented if she had spoken up about the omitted fire-safety checklist. But then she remembers an obstetric hemorrhage years ago, where she was shouted at for calling for blood. Traumatized, she learned to keep quiet, but since the operating room fire, she has felt powerless and anxious. She has been wondering about whether this is the right job for her and has not been sleeping well.

A few additional questions:

- How do traumatic learning experiences undermine a patient safety culture?
- What injuries can a health care professional suffer when morally conflicted?
- Is this burnout or something else? How is Nurse Corage's response different from others?

Burnout/Wellness vs Moral Injury/Resilience

- **Burnout syndrome** comprises emotional exhaustion, depersonalization, and diminished sense of personal accomplishment; it can arise from myriad drivers, may differ between genders, and can be magnified after a patient safety event.
- **Wellness** is an active process through which people become aware of, and make choices toward, optimal health and vitality, encompassing physical, emotional, intellectual, spiritual, interpersonal, social and environmental well-being.
- **Moral Injury** is damage to one's conscience or moral compass when that person witnesses, perpetrates, or fails to prevent acts that transgress one's own moral beliefs, values, or ethical codes of conducts. It may involve self-betrayal of one's own code, but especially involving betrayal of principles by those with authority.
- **Moral distress** is an emotional state that arises when a person feels compelled to take actions that diverge from what is felt to be ethically correct. It is often associated with a sense of powerlessness, anxiety, or depression.
- **Moral resilience** is the internal capacity to restore and sustain their personal integrity in response to moral adversity; a related concept is moral courage that involves strength to speak up despite the fear of repercussions.

Fig. 8. Comparison of burnout, wellness, moral injury, and moral resilience.

What Is Moral Suffering and Injury?

Moral trauma is distinct from burnout and is increasingly being recognized as an important factor affecting health care professionals[30] (**Fig. 8**). It involves anguish from witnessing, perpetrating, or failing to prevent events that transgress deeply held moral beliefs—as when individuals are rushed and fail to comply with safety practices.[31] Moral suffering is defined as "anguish experienced in response to moral harms, wrongs, or failures and unrelieved moral stress."[32] It represents a continuum, wherein the initial inciting event induces a state of emotional discomfort (ie, moral distress) and recurrent insults or failure to resolve a single powerful incident progresses to moral injury. Nurse Corage, who wishes to model transparency, finds herself in a morally conflicted situation: not only is she distressed that family is not receiving the whole story, but she has no confidence that Dr Scalpelle's chair will ever know the truth. Even if his chair gets the facts, can he handle the truth?

After a patient is harmed, moral wounds often emerge. Members of the team may have felt unable to speak up or take actions when an unsafe work environment emerged; they may have ongoing compunction from inability to speak honestly and openly with patients or families about what transpired. Situations that betray one's moral convictions can imperil integrity and well-being (**Fig. 9**), and 1 in 3 clinicians

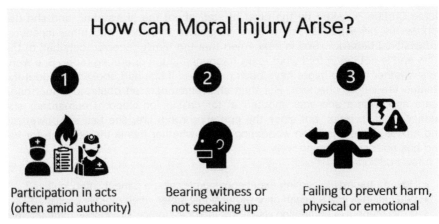

How can Moral Injury Arise?

1 — Participation in acts (often amid authority)

2 — Bearing witness or not speaking up

3 — Failing to prevent harm, physical or emotional

Fig. 9. Causes of moral injury.

reports symptoms of moral injury.[32] Inner dissonance may occur when a health care professional feels unable to address ongoing needs of the patient and family, cannot offer sincere apology, or is unable to restore trust. When learners are trained in disclosure, they lose these skills if their faculty role models are not transparent,[33] perpetuating generations of hiding truths and continuing moral injury.

Moral injury only became widely recognized in medicine in 2018,[27] and until 2020 no valid instrument existed to quantify moral injury in health care professionals.[34] In the COVID-19 era, the moral conflicts relating to resource shortages greatly increased both prevalence and awareness of moral injury. Because moral injury is often associated with perceived betrayals by those in authority, leadership responses are vitally important. Systems aimed at fostering a "just" culture require the infrastructure to support ethical practice, and the 2 must be aligned to achieve synergistic effects and ensure sustainability. Furthermore, experiences of microaggression, verbal abuse, and violence can also jeopardize relational integrity and undermine professional morale and sense of meaning.

How Can the Culture of Health Care Predispose to Moral Injury?

Moral injury is often perpetrated by systems. For example, *Deny-and-defend* responses to patient harm cast patients as adversaries—something that is deeply demoralizing to empathic professionals; it devalues what attracted them to patient care. Broken trust among team members can cause clinicians to doubt themselves, their intentions, and their humanity—losing connection with their core purpose. Thinking and acting in ways that are incongruent with one's professional code of ethics erodes personal and relational integrity. Clinicians may lose joy and meaning in their work. Some perseverate or isolate; others become hardened and cynical. When moral distress is a prominent feature, symptoms of shame, guilt, anger, and powerlessness often dominate, often accompanied by anxiety, depression, and poor sleep.[35]

The risk of moral injury escalates when unprofessional behaviors persist, as when leadership casts a blind eye on a disrespectful surgeon who brings significant resources to the organization. Power imbalances between clinicians are reinforced when the response of nonphysicians is dismissed, when complaints fail to translate into definitive action, or when actions are inequitably applied. For example, what would happen to a nurse who behaved similarly to Dr Scalpelle? Likely there would be prompt disciplinary action and perhaps termination; fear of retaliation is very real. Teamwork can become dysfunctional as lapses of integrity become tolerated or normalized—allowing patient care to deteriorate and missing an opportunity to address the moral wounds that can arise from such situations.

This relationship between unprofessional behavior and moral trauma is seldom acknowledged, but the transgressions are cumulative, and each one breaks trust. When trust is broken, people start to doubt themselves and others—they become disconnected from what matters most to them. When these aspects are silenced, the moral residue that accumulates over time can be substantial and corrosive. For example, if risk management tells Nurse Corage, "Don't talk to anyone," gossip inevitably begins to create an alternate narrative that breaks trust among the team. People begin to doubt their own competence and basic goodness. They begin to ask—Am I still a good person? Am I still a good clinician? In any of these situations, clinicians may spiral into guilt and shame. Many clinicians experience guilt that is misplaced or that is out of proportion to the individual's role. These observations highlight the interdependency of patient care and caregiver wellness and professionalism (**Fig. 10**).

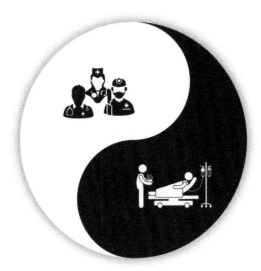

Fig. 10. Interdependency of patient care and caregiver wellness and professionalism.

When leadership is unresponsive, Dr Scalpelle's disruptive behaviors in the operating room and the subsequent operating room fire—where a flammable alcohol-based prep ignited in a high oxygen field—can be framed in perverse ways. Nurse Corage, a steadfast professional, performed the surgical prep in accordance with trusted practices—but without benefit of the guidance she requested from Dr Scalpelle. Tragically, she is at high risk for self-doubt in a system that tolerates Dr Scalpelle's behavior and may even find herself in the cross hairs for using a flammable prep. Yet, it was Dr Scalpelle who set into motion the chain of events that led to the fire: the oxygen flow dialed up under duress; the rebuffing of Nurse Corage as she sought guidance on the surgical prep; the pressure to rush and skip the fire safety checklist; the chilling effect of an intolerant surgeon on the team's ability to stop the line—"pulling the Andon cord" in the language of quality improvement to halt activity for a problem; and Dr Scalpelle's impetuous cauterization that was the proximal cause for oxygen and alcohol to catch flame.

Shame focuses on the appraisal of what others think of us, is often prominent in these situations, and can be intensified when the "cone of silence" prevents individuals and groups from processing what has happened in a psychologically safe environment. The rigidity of health care roles coupled with the cultural expectation to "not make waves" and power differentials can intensify the distress that clinicians experience. Physical sensations or symptoms are often perceived before one is cognizant of inner dissonance.[36–38] Individuals may perceive inability to resolve the ethical quandary as a personal moral failing. When moral distress is recurring or unresolved it can overwhelm a person's reparative and coping capacity, progressing to moral injury, which can erode sense of worth and damage a person's humanity. As exemplified by the vignette, moral injury can arise from acts of commission or omission, including witnessing a fellow team member who puts a patient in harm's way. Moral injury may prompt individuals to question their moral compass or that of the entire profession.[39]

How Can Moral Resilience Protect From Moral Injury?

Moral resilience is the internal capacity to restore and sustain their personal integrity in response to moral injury.[30] The capacities of moral resilience are shown in **Fig. 11**. It is

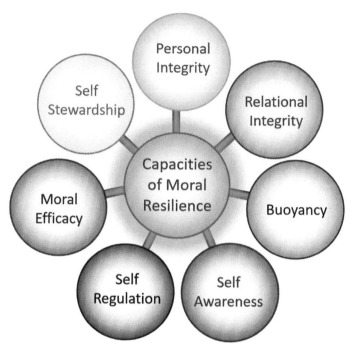

Fig. 11. Capacities of moral resilience.

oriented toward facing the challenges instead of turning away from them and requires knowing who we are and what we stand for in our life and work, while appreciating our own limitations. Courage is the engine of integrity to do the right thing even when there is risk or resistance. When faced with hard choices, integrity connects us to our core values and can motivate integrity preserving action.

Cultivating moral resilience is a promising strategy for countering moral adversity and burnout. With refinement of validated research tools, including development of the Rushton Moral Resilience Scale,[40] a more nuanced understanding has emerged of moral resilience, its associations, and how it can be fostered. The moral resilience scale has 4 subdomains (Responses to Moral Adversity, Personal Integrity, Moral Efficacy, and Relational Integrity). Higher moral resilience is associated with lower overall levels of burnout and reduced turnover intention. Furthermore, moral resilience is a protective resource to mitigate the detrimental effects of both moral distress and moral injury.

When an individual has insight into his own moral sufferings, he can identify strategies that will restore integrity, particularly when leadership is responsive to systemic contributors to the distress. Just as it is necessary to identify the root factors that contributed to a medical error, organizations must similarly create surveillance systems to identify lapses in integrity and ethical practice and put in place mechanisms to address them. Furthermore, because moral resilience factors may be modifiable, addressing its subcomponents may afford an opportunity for interventions conducive to growth and empowerment when morally injurious situations are encountered in clinical settings. Because validated measurement of subdomains of moral resilience has

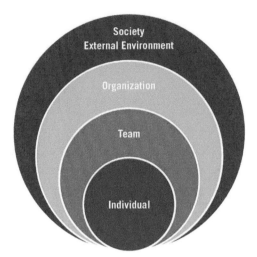

Fig. 12. A socioecological perspective emphasizes that resilience does not reside solely in the individual. Just as burnout and moral distress arise from a complex interplay of individual and systemic factors, so too does the adaptive response for resilience. (*From* Davidson P, Rushton CH, Kurtz M, et al J Clin Nurs. 2018 Mar;27(5-6); also: Pappas S, Rushton CH. Designing Resilience into the Work Environment. In: High Reliability Organizations, 2nd ed. Ed. Oster CA and Braaten JS. Sigma Theta Tau International Honor Society of Nursing. 2021. Indianapolis, IN; with permission.)

become more nuanced, the protective effects of moral resilience on both turnover intent and burnout are becoming more evident. Such findings are particularly important in the face of increasing levels of burnout and escalating clinician shortages.

A socioecological lens can add nuance to understanding how moral resilience relates to the ethical challenges encountered by health professionals in the context of their daily work (**Fig. 12**). Increasingly, health care professionals are confronted with ethical dilemmas that span interpersonal, sociopolitical, cultural, economic, and health care operational domains.[41] Often, ethical concepts are introduced in an abstract manner that lacks the practical basis necessary to translate such teachings into safe, equitable, and high-quality patient care. Leadership buy-in and stakeholder engagement are necessary to address situations where legal or regulatory processes

---

Key Characteristics of Moral Resilience

- Cultivating mindfulness to support focus and clarity of mind
- Learning to self-regulate to disrupt negative patterns of thinking and behaving
- Developing self-awareness and insight
- Deepening moral sensitivity
- Discerning ethical challenges and principled actions
- Nurturing the willingness to take courageous action
- Preserving one's integrity, as well as the integrity of the team, and others

Fig. 13. Moral resilience characteristics. (*Adapted from* Rushton CH. Cultivating Moral Resilience. Am J Nurs. 2017 Feb;117(2 Suppl 1):S11-S15. https://doi.org/10.1097/01.NAJ. 0000512205.93596.00. PMID: 28085701; with permission.)

may cause misalignment with ethical precepts. Ethical decision-making and practice are intertwined, and organizational efforts that allow clinicians to articulate concerns, reconcile inconsistencies, and practice in accordance with their moral code can minimize moral distress.

Fig. 13 summarizes strategies for harnessing the resilient capacity of clinicians, which protect against the deleterious effects of moral adversity.[42] At the core of moral resilience is recognizing the importance of integrity and adopting practices that support moral rectitude in actions and self-awareness around ethical dilemmas and conflict such as those outlined in the case example. Moral resilience involves cultivating mindfulness, learning to disrupt negative thought patterns, deepening moral sensitivity, identifying ethical challenges, finding the strength to take courageous action, and preserving personal integrity. Ongoing work is illuminating how subdomains of moral resilience and burnout relate to one another.

Moral resilience is not the exclusive responsibility of clinicians—leaders have a responsibility to create the conditions for integrity to thrive. Leaders must create systems that support routinely doing the right thing, without requiring a heroic act. Individual moral resilience strategies must be coupled with systemic investments that ensure a just culture. Leaders should strive to understand moral suffering, develop approaches to identify it, and implement strategies that afford relief to those experiencing it.

How Does Collective Resilience Strengthen a Team and Organization?

Collective resilience captures the interconnectedness of human experience; it allows us to pool collective strength and plumb greater depths of our collective character

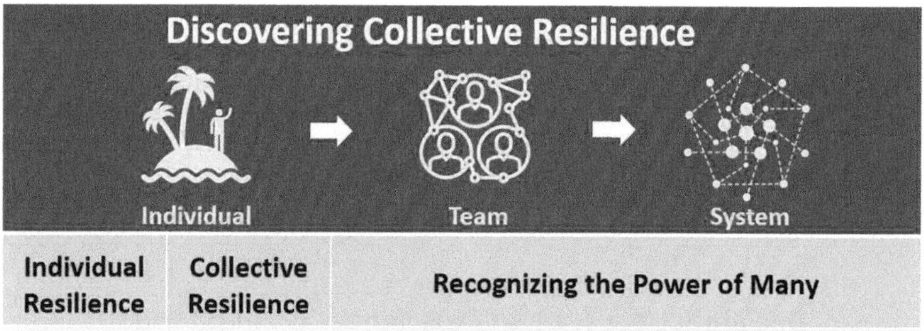

Individual Resilience	Collective Resilience	Recognizing the Power of Many
Walks Alone	Partners	When resilience resides solely in the individual, it is siloed; it walk alone when facing challenges. Collective resilience partners, creating interconnected teams, units, and systems.
Shields	Adapts	Individual resilience shields a person from acute shocks; but collective resilience adds the dynamic adaptive capacity that allow for sustainable solutions in new conditions.
Radiates	Imbues	Resilient individuals radiate energy in the face of adversity; collective resilience also imbues the team with shared purpose, recognizing the commonality of human experience.
Taps	Pools	Individuals tap a finite reservoir of resilience; cohesive teams can pool their resilience, drawing on a deeper well fed by many streams so they can withstand more destabilizing stresses.

Fig. 14. Comparison of individual versus collective resilience.

(**Fig. 14**), but it requires trust, respect, and teamwork. Simply addressing burnout is a low bar, as many professionals are drawn to improving the lives of others and see their work as a calling.[43] A more appropriate goal is achieving professional fulfillment, recognizing that the care of patients and promoting wellness of the team are interdependent, as the human experience reciprocally affects all stakeholders.[1] Similarly, naming the moral aspects of these situations opens new avenues to design specific interventions to address them.

Attention to creating psychologically safe spaces for interprofessional teams to learn from safety near misses and errors and lapses in integrity offer structural means for shifting the culture. Linking physician well-being to safety and quality metrics may help in prioritizing physician wellness.[21] Occupational well-being is no longer solely about the individual physician, as malpractice carriers and organizations may realize economic advantages from promoting professional fulfillment and taking steps to mitigate work exhaustion, interpersonal disengagement, and moral injury. There is a growing realization that resilience often does not reside solely in the individual. Elevating human experience in health care allows for better experiences and outcomes for patients while achieving a more rewarding collaborative environment for health care professionals. This realization has led to a Declaration for Human Experience (**Fig. 15**).

How Do We Help Professionals Find the Road to Recovery?

Systems must be designed with intentionality so that professionals get the help that they need. If Dr Scalpelle continues to engage in risky behaviors, then Nurse Corage and other team members must be empowered to act. Suppose Dr Scalpelle routinely refuses to honor time-outs, citing increased surgical volumes, productivity pressures, and slow turnover. How should the team respond? The reporting system plays a critical role in documenting concerns. Suppose Dr Scalpelle says, "It's *impossible* to go through the meaningless exercise every case... I have *never* had a wrong site procedure. I'm leaving. Page me when we're ready to start." In the face of such obstinacy, the system allows the team to hold the line on safety. And in doing so, the team supports wellness; everyone—including the patient—needs to be able to stop the line, as part of our collective commitment to professional accountability.[44]

Declaration for Human Experience Commitments

- Acknowledge and dismantle systemic racism and prejudice, tackle disparities and provide the highest-quality, most equitable care possible.
- Understand and act on the needs and vulnerabilities of the healthcare workforce to honor their commitment and reaffirm and reenergize their purpose.
- Recognize and maintain a focus on what matters most to patients, their family members and care partners to ensure unparalleled care and a commitment to health and well-being.
- Collaborate through shared learning within and between organizations, systems and the broader healthcare continuum to forge a bold new path to a more human-centered, equitable and effective healthcare system.

Fig. 15. Tenets of the declaration of human experience. (*Adapted from* theberylinstitute.org/news/562365/Declaration-for-Human-Experience-Calls-for-Transformation-of-Healthcare.htm.; with permission.)

CASE EXAMPLE (CONTINUED)

In response to Nurse Corage's account of the operating room fire, the Chief Medical Officer investigates Dr Scalpelle's role in disrupting team dynamics. Review of unsolicited patient and coworker grievances reveals a theme of lack of respect for patients, policies, and fellow professionals. Dr Propofal, who has worked with Dr Scalpelle for many years, serves as a peer messenger. Back from sabbatical, she takes Dr Scalpelle to lunch and shares the data on complaints and observations. Dr Scalpelle remains impassive, and 2 weeks later another unsolicited patient complaint arrives, reporting that Dr Scalpelle ridiculed them. The department chair directs Dr Scalpelle to a program for professional help. Indignant, Dr Scalpelle exclaims, "I AM NOT GOING."

When Dr Scalpelle refuses help, he also turns his back on the team. The tiered interventions move him to the next level of a guided intervention. Although he has failed to self-regulate, he has a choice — he can either accept help and work toward rejoining the professional community or he can take another step toward departure from clinical care. For most of the individuals, the tiered approach empowers the clinician to modify their behavior so they can resume serving the clinical mission. Such is the case for Dr Scalpelle, in this case.

Leaders have a duty to create psychological safety and accountability, and in doing so they foster wellness and resilience. It is this safety that prevents an airway fire—because Dr Scalpelle fully participates in the operating room time-out; if he does not pause, then Nurse Corage's trust in the system motivates her to report, setting into motion the accountability machinery. Coffee is served and, if that does not suffice, then tiered interventions follow—an approach now used across

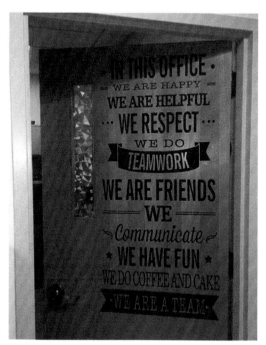

Fig. 16. Shared office at Michigan Medicine, bringing together educators, leads, and managers.

hundreds of institutions. Even in unsafe cultures, one sometimes finds the rare, shining light who will speak out at great risk or become a whistle blower; but it should not require heroic courage to do what is right. Tiered systems have achieved sustained success in improving adherence to hand hygiene, antibiotic stewardship, and vaccine compliance; reducing surgical site infections; and addressing physicians with high malpractice claims risk.[27,45,46] The resulting accountability restores team trust and joy in work.

In the pursuit of occupational wellness and resilience in health care, leaders must provide professionals the help they need. Dr Scalpelle is connected to skilled professionals that work with him to address long-neglected mental illness; he also receives coaching that empowers him to develop a capacity for self-regulation and eventually allows him to rejoin his professional colleagues. Dr Propofal engages in an employee wellness program that restores her joy in teaching, research, and patient care. Drs Resedent and Lerner are offered counseling and flexibility in their residency training program, which allows recovery from traumatic learning experiences and return to a path of excellence in clinical care. The patient and family are attended to with solicitude, and trust begins to be restored. Finally, Nurse Corage recovers from her moral injury as transparency is achieved with the family and as professional accountability restored, once again bringing her work into alignment with her moral center.

SUMMARY

We share a responsibility to take decisive measures to alleviate burnout, address moral adversity, and achieve integrity and collective resilience. Doing so requires bold leadership initiatives and grassroots efforts. When the Institute of Medicine issued *To Err is Human,*[24] it ushered in the modern patient safety movement with an emphasis on building safer systems. Two decades later, we recognize a second truth that *To Care is Human*[47]—that embracing shared human experience and assuring well-being of health care professional is a moral imperative. Restoring meaning, purpose, and joy in work is vital to our professional identity and is necessary for safe, effective, and morally grounded care. A culture of accountability characterized by honesty, transparency, and integrity is indispensable to creating an inviting workplace—one where the door to teamwork is always open and all are valued when they enter (**Fig. 16**).

REFERENCES

1. Trockel M, Bohman B, Lesure E, et al. A brief instrument to assess both burnout and professional fulfillment in physicians: reliability and validity, including correlation with self-reported medical errors, in a sample of resident and practicing physicians. Acad Psychiatry 2018;42(1):11–24.
2. National Academies of Sciences, Engineering, and Medicine. Taking action against clinician burnout: a systems approach to professional well-being. Washington (DC): The National Academies Press; 2019. https://doi.org/10.17226/25521. Available at:.
3. Weiner K. Clinician burnout is only getting worse. Here's how to tackle the problem. NEJM Catalyst Innov Care Deliv 2021;2(2):1–21.
4. Panagioti M, Geraghty K, Johnson J, et al. Association between physician burnout and patient safety, professionalism, and patient satisfaction: a systematic review and meta-analysis. JAMA Intern Med 2018;178(10):1317–31.
5. Shanafelt T, Goh J, Sinsky C. The business case for investing in physician well-being. JAMA Intern Med 2017;177(12):1826–32.

6. Shanafelt TD, Mungo M, Schmitgen J, et al. Longitudinal study evaluating the association between physician burnout and changes in professional work effort. Mayo Clin Proc 2016;91(4):422–31.

7. Sinsky CA, Dyrbye LN, West CP, et al. Professional satisfaction and the career plans of US physicians. Mayo Clin Proc 2017;92(11):1625–35.

8. Hamidi MS, Bohman B, Sandborg C, et al. Estimating institutional physician turnover attributable to self-reported burnout and associated financial burden: a case study. BMC Health Serv Res 2018;18(1):851.

9. Windover AK, Martinez K, Mercer MB, et al. Correlates and outcomes of physician burnout within a large academic medical center. JAMA Intern Med 2018;178(6):856–8.

10. Leiter MP, Maslach C. Nurse turnover: the mediating role of burnout. J Nurs Manag 2009;17(3):331–9.

11. Melnyk BM. Burnout, depression and suicide in nurses/clinicians and learners: an urgent call for action to enhance professional well-being and healthcare safety. Worldviews Evid Based Nurs 2020;17(1):2–5.

12. Poncet MC, Toullic P, Papazian L, et al. Burnout syndrome in critical care nursing staff. Am J Respir Crit Care Med 2007;175(7):698–704.

13. Klein J, Grosse Frie K, Blum K, et al. Burnout and perceived quality of care among German clinicians in surgery. Int J Qual Health Care 2010;22(6):525–30.

14. Kuerer HM, Eberlein TJ, Pollock RE, et al. Career satisfaction, practice patterns and burnout among surgical oncologists: report on the quality of life of members of the Society of Surgical Oncology. Ann Surg Oncol 2007;14(11):3043–53.

15. Shanafelt TD, Balch CM, Bechamps G, et al. Burnout and medical errors among American surgeons. Ann Surg 2010;251(6):995–1000.

16. Shanafelt TD, Gradishar WJ, Kosty M, et al. Burnout and career satisfaction among US oncologists. J Clin Oncol 2014;32(7):678–86.

17. Wallace JE, Lemaire J. Physician well being and quality of patient care: an exploratory study of the missing link. Psychol Health Med 2009;14(5):545–52.

18. Thompson DM, Brenner MJ. Prescribing time to temporize burnout: are we hacking at the branches, or striking at the root? JAMA Otolaryngol Head Neck Surg 2020;146(2):103–5.

19. Catron TF, Guillamondegui OD, Karrass J, et al. Patient complaints and adverse surgical outcomes. Am J Med Qual 2016;31(5):415–22.

20. Cooper WO, Guillamondegui O, Hines OJ, et al. Use of unsolicited patient observations to identify surgeons with increased risk for postoperative complications. JAMA Surg 2017;152(6):522–9.

21. Hickson GB, Federspiel CF, Pichert JW, et al. Patient complaints and malpractice risk. JAMA 2002;287(22):2951–7.

22. Fahrenkopf AM, Sectish TC, Barger LK, et al. Rates of medication errors among depressed and burnt out residents: prospective cohort study. BMJ 2008;336(7642):488–91.

23. Halbesleben JR, Rathert C. Linking physician burnout and patient outcomes: exploring the dyadic relationship between physicians and patients. Health Care Manage Rev 2008;33(1):29–39.

24. Institute of Medicine (US) Committee on Quality of Health Care in America Linda T. Kohn, Janet M. Corrigan, Molla S. Donaldson, editors. To err is human: building a safer health system. Washington, D.C.: National Academies Press; 2000.

25. Hickson GBM, I.N., Pichert JW, et al. Balancing systems and individual accountability in a safety culture. Chapter 1. In: From front office to front line. Essential

issues for healthcare leaders. 2nd edition. Oakbrook Terrace (IL): Joint Commission Resources; 2012.

26. Cooper WO, Spain DA, Guillamondegui O, et al. Association of coworker reports about unprofessional behavior by surgeons with surgical complications in their patients. JAMA Surg 2019;154(9):828–34.

27. Talbot TR, Johnson JG, Fergus C, et al. Sustained improvement in hand hygiene adherence: utilizing shared accountability and financial incentives. Infect Control Hosp Epidemiol 2013;34(11):1129–36.

28. Rushton CH. Moral resilience: a capacity for navigating moral distress in critical care. AACN Adv Crit Care 2016;27(1):111–9.

29. Truog RD, Campbell ML, Curtis JR, et al. Recommendations for end-of-life care in the intensive care unit: a consensus statement by the American College [corrected] of Critical Care Medicine. Crit Care Med 2008;36(3):953–63.

30. Rushton CH. Conceptualizing moral resilience. In: Rushton CH, editor. Moral resilience: transforming moral suffering. Oxford: Oxford University Press; 2018. p. 125–49.

31. Litz BTS N, Delaney E, Lebowitz L, et al. Moral injury and moral repair in war Veterans: A preliminary model and intervention strategy. Clin Psychol Rev 2009; 29(8):695–706.

32. Rushton CH, Rushton CH. Mapping the path of moral adversity. In: CH R, editor. Moral resilience: transforming moral suffering in healthcare. New York: Oxford University Press; 2018. p. 52–76.

33. Martinez W, Lehmann LS, Thomas EJ, et al. Speaking up about traditional and professionalism-related patient safety threats: a national survey of interns and residents. BMJ Qual Saf 2017;26(11):869–80.

34. Tong Y, Wang Z, Sun Y, et al. Psychometric properties of the chinese version of short-form community attitudes toward mentally illness scale in medical students and primary healthcare workers. Front Psychiatry 2020;11:337.

35. Rushton CH, Turner K, Brock RN, et al. Invisible moral wounds of the COVID-19 pandemic: are we experiencing moral injury? AACN Adv Crit Care 2021;32(1): 119–25.

36. Burston AS, Tuckett AG. Moral distress in nursing: contributing factors, outcomes and interventions. Nurs Ethics 2013;20(3):312–24.

37. Hanna DR. The lived experience of moral distress: nurses who assisted with elective abortions. Res Theor Nurs Pract 2005;19(1):95–124.

38. Rushton CH, Kaszniak AW, Halifax JS. A framework for understanding moral distress among palliative care clinicians. J Palliat Med 2013;16(9):1074–9.

39. Dean W, Talbot SG, Caplan A. Clarifying the language of clinician distress. JAMA 2020;323(10):923–4.

40. Heinze KE, Hanson G, Holtz H, et al. Measuring health care interprofessionals' moral resilience: validation of the rushton moral resilience scale. J Palliat Med 2021;24(6):865–72.

41. Davidson P, Rushton CH, Kurtz M, et al. A social-ecological framework: a model for addressing ethical practice in nursing. J Clin Nurs 2018;27(5–6):e1233–41.

42. Rushton CH. Designing sustainable systems for ethical practice. In: Rushton CH, editor. Moral resilience: transforming moral suffering in healthcare. Oxford: Oxford University Press; 2018. p. 206–42.

43. Yoon JD, Daley BM, Curlin FA. The association between a sense of calling and physician well-being: a National Study of Primary Care Physicians and Psychiatrists. Acad Psychiatry 2017;41(2):167–73.

44. Bell SK, Martinez W. Every patient should be enabled to stop the line. BMJ Qual Saf 2019;28(3):172–6.
45. Hickson GB, Pichert JW, Webb LE, et al. A complementary approach to promoting professionalism: identifying, measuring, and addressing unprofessional behaviors. Acad Med 2007;82(11):1040–8.
46. Pichert JW, Moore IN, Hickson GB. Professionals promoting professionalism. Jt Comm J Qual Patient Saf 2011;37(10):446.
47. Dzau VJ, Kirch DG, Nasca TJ. To care is human - collectively confronting the clinician-burnout crisis. N Engl J Med 2018;378(4):312–4.

Making the Business Case for Quality and Safety

Rahul K. Shah, MD, MBA*, Richelle Reinhart, MD, Jessica Cronin, MD, MBA

KEYWORDS

- Safety • Quality • Business • Management • Outcomes • Return on investment
- Financial statements • Health care

KEY POINTS

- Quality and safety have evolved to require a business case to support continued investments in this crucial work.
- Leaders and managers must use financial tools based on objective data coupled with subjective storytelling to make a compelling business case.
- The top health care organizations continue to invest in quality and safety and have evolved by developing robust structures to support continued efforts to deliver the highest-quality care for patients and families.
- Investing in quality and safety efforts is financially and morally the right decision with expenditures paying off in the long term through tangible and intangible returns.
- In the future, health care organizations will need an individual with a strong financial background on its multidisciplinary Quality and Safety team.

INTRODUCTION/HISTORY/DEFINITIONS/BACKGROUND

Quality and safety are not new concepts in American health care; they are tenets of modern medicine. A lone voice, Earnest Avery Codman, was a trailblazer in the mid-twentieth century advocating for systems to track patient outcomes in order to look back and assess what went well and what failed. His work was the predecessor of the Joint Commission and hence began a phase in modern medicine focused on ensuring that care delivery is both quasi-standardized and of the highest quality in the safest manner.

A second tipping point occurred at the turn of the century (1999–2000) with the Institute of Medicine's landmark report, "To Err is Human."[1] This report alerted modern medicine and acted as a clarion call to do better and how to do better with regards to safety. As expected, there was public outcry that change and transparency were necessary, with an explosion of work stemming from the seminal piece. A panoply

The authors have nothing to disclose.

George Washington University School of Health Sciences, Children's National Hospital, 5th Floor, West Wing, Suite 403, 111 Michigan Avenue, Northwest, Washington, DC 20010, USA
* Corresponding author.
E-mail address: rshah@childrensnational.org

Otolaryngol Clin N Am 55 (2022) 105–113
https://doi.org/10.1016/j.otc.2021.07.008
0030-6665/22/© 2021 Elsevier Inc. All rights reserved.

of regulatory initiatives were rolled out in efforts to combat latent safety defects and perceived system flaws, and there was the beginning of nurses, doctors, and medical staff's owning the responsibility of policing bad clinicians (peer review become robust, and this was supported by accreditation organizations like the Joint Commission and their concepts of on-going professional practice evaluations and focused professional practice evaluations).

For providers, hospitals, and health care organizations, we consider the early part of the twenty–first century as the inflection point for safety and quality. No longer was safety and quality hidden at the management level; Boards placed outcomes at the top of the agenda. Boards opened their meetings with patient safety stories as a technique to connect disparate members to the mission of the organization under their governance. As Boards embraced the inherent value in promoting quality and safety, management followed and operationalized their Boards governance.

Soon after the 2000s, health care managers and leaders quickly realized that to deliver on the public's and the Board's expectations of the highest possible quality of care delivered in the safest manner, they needed to increase their capacity and capability of their employees. The leap in American health care with regards to quality and safety could not occur in isolation. The avalanche of initiatives following the Institute of Medicine's report greatly helped accelerate health care leaders and managers to embrace the change and drive the work in their organizations because of 1 simple fact: *a business case can be made for the work*.

Because of alignment of regulatory mandates, legislative incentives, and payer (insurance) support, health care organizations had the requisite funding to perform work to increase their capacity (organizational and individual time/resources to embark on quality improvement initiatives) and capability (the know-how for organizations and individuals to perform the work of improvement).

Before the 2000s, most in American health care realized that quality and safety were important. This apathetic sentiment rapidly changed in the past 2 decades to a prevailing understanding that not only is quality and safety the right thing to do but also there exists a financial case and as such the sentiment now is: "It makes financial sense *and* is the right thing to do." This duality makes advocating and promoting quality and safety initiatives not a complete uphill battle if the advocate uses basic business principles.

For health care directors to be agile in making the business case for their quality and safety efforts, they must have a basic understanding of accounting and finance. A manager or leader that does not have this background must partner with a business-minded individual in their organization so they can be owners of the initiative as a dyad. Without a business lens, a quality and safety initiative will not be able to garner the full attention necessary to accelerate improvement and achieve completion.

There are 3 financial statements that reflect an organization's financial performance that health care leaders should be aware of: income statement, balance sheet, and cash flow statement. An income statement tells the story of a business's revenue and costs. Revenue and costs are generally accounted for in the specific time period in which they are incurred. Most common sources of revenue for hospitals are payment for patient care services by private insurance companies and the government (Centers for Medicare and Medicaid). The largest hospital expenses are payroll, administrative, and supplies costs. The income statement shows the net income of an organization by subtracting costs from revenue. However, health care organizations often use metrics other than net income to understand profitability. Earnings before interest and taxes or earnings before interest, taxes, depreciation, and amortization are frequently used to better understand earnings achieved from its operations because these metrics exclude noncash line items (depreciation and amortization) and items (interest and taxes) that can fluctuate year to year for reasons unrelated to operations. These metrics can elucidate an organization's profitability, which, for most hospitals, are razor thin margins. A health care leader can use the income statement to understand which business lines are the most profitable and which business areas are growing; this information is crucial to place a quality and safety initiative in perspective for the organization.

A statement of cash flow reflects how cash is made and spent by the organization over a specific period of time. Three different sections of the cash flow statement include operations, investments, and financing. Operating cash flow includes cash received through the sales of products or services. The sale or purchase of property, plant, and equipment or other capital expenditures will be accounted for in the investments section of the cash flow statement. The financing section reflects the flow of cash between an organization and its creditors (change in debt) as well as its shareholders (change in equity). Although the cash flow statement is not often specifically referenced, quality and safety leaders must understand which business areas are sources of cash for the hospital system and how their initiatives may potentially impact how cash flows through the organization.

Third, the balance sheet tells the story of a business's assets (what it owns) and liabilities (what it owes) in a certain moment in time. In a for-profit company, the difference between assets and liabilities is shareholders' equity, or what the company is worth to its owners if all assets were sold and all liabilities were paid off. Nonprofit organizations do not have shareholders, so this difference is called net assets. For example, if an organization takes out a loan of $10,000 from a bank, then liabilities go up by $10,000 and assets (in the form of cash) go up by $10,000, whereas shareholders' equity does not change. Organizations use line items within balance sheets to create ratios that reflect aspects of its financial health, including liquidity (amount of liquid assets like cash an organization has relative to less-liquid assets like a building) and leverage (amount of debt an organization has to finance its operations). Ratios can also be calculated using multiple financial statements to understand aspects like returns on investments (ROI). ROI is a way to measure the value or financial gains created by an intervention, taking into account the initial investment required. It is also a metric that allows health care leaders to compare possible interventions and decide which investments to prioritize. Of course, there are other more sophisticated measures (net present value, and so forth) that are beyond the scope of this review article.

The case for telehealth during the COVID-19 pandemic is an example of how an investment can make financial sense with a compelling ROI and is the right thing to do. When the pandemic began, revenue for hospitals dropped dramatically as demand for in-person clinic visits, emergency room visits, elective operations, and other revenue-generating services decreased. At the same time, because many hospital costs are fixed and cannot be reduced in the short term, profitability plummeted. Hospital leaders quickly identified alternative revenue sources like telehealth, which was compulsory to provide care for their patients. Other factors also played a role, increasing demand for telehealth. The regulatory environment became more favorable, as it was easier to be reimbursed for telehealth visits, and there was increased patient and provider interest. Most importantly, telehealth ensured hospitals could provide patients safe access to the care they need. In a few short months, the ROI for a robust telehealth platform changed dramatically, and the business case for telehealth was clear. Telehealth became a relatively low-cost investment that generated significant revenue for many hospital systems and is likely to be a permanent care delivery format postpandemic. Such successes during the COVID-19 pandemic illustrate how financial tools can help build a business case to improve delivery of high-quality care in a changing environment.

NATURE OF THE PROBLEM

As the prior section described, there is tremendous public, Board, and organizational attention toward quality and safety outcomes. This attention is worldwide; in 2019, the World Health Organization created a call to action for patient safety. Their memo reminded health care organizations internationally that the focus should remain on patient-centered care with an emphasis on safety culture. They noted that harm from hospital-acquired conditions is known to be a top 10 cause of death and compared these numbers with other worldwide crises, such as mortality from tuberculosis and malaria.[2]

The business case for telehealth showed that this investment not only was the right thing to do to improve patient access to care but also had a compelling ROI with a clear positive impact on revenue. However, quality and safety initiatives are rarely revenue-generating, and there is significant pressure on hospitals to control costs given their narrow profitability. Nevertheless, as Berwick and Cassel argue,[3] investment in quality and safety processes is the best way to control costs. Therefore, it is critical for quality and safety leaders to prove beneficial financial impact downstream to compel the organization to continue to invest in safe, high-quality care.

Downstream financial benefits from quality and safety projects are usually in the form of cost savings. For example, some insurance companies will not reimburse a health care organization if a patient develops a hospital-acquired condition. This makes intuitive sense, as the insurer wants to ensure their member is receiving the best care, and a hospital-acquired condition implies a deviation from high-quality care. However, for the health care organization, payment denial for care for an expensive admission can be devastating. For example, using business lexicon, analysis, and strategies, health care organizational leaders and managers must be able to demonstrate that a $25,000 investment in a quality improvement project based in the intensive care unit with a specific aim to reduce the rate of central line associated blood stream infections (CLABSIs) from 2.7 to 2.3 in 6 months and sustain for a year will easily be recouped by saving "x" number of CLABSIs. The peer-reviewed literature has started becoming filled with articles demonstrating the "costs" of hospital-acquired conditions.

Similar to hospital-acquired conditions, some insurance companies will not reimburse a health care organization for a patient's hospital stay if the patient gets readmitted to the hospital within 30 days of being discharged. Quality and safety initiatives that reduce readmissions are also compelling investments for health care organizations.

Lawsuits arising from potentially avoidable serious adverse events within a hospital system can also be costly, particularly in the setting of self-insured health care organizations. Consistent reduction in serious adverse events not only reduces out of pocket for the hospital but also reduces reinsurance premiums.[4]

We have described at length the direct cost benefits of saving a hospital from readmission costs, health care-acquired conditions, lawsuits, and insurance payment denials. There are also more intangible benefits to improving the quality of a hospital's care. For example, the positive reputation of a hospital that consistently ranks highly in patient safety is indisputable. This recognition will then bring more reputable professionals and perhaps improved scientific output, again pushing the organization higher in its rankings. Multiple studies have shown the beneficial impact of a hospital publicly reporting its achievements, along with a positive relationship between the public's perception and a hospital's performance. Consumers (patients) will continue to show their support for these high-ranking hospitals by choosing to obtain their care there. These indirect benefits cannot be ignored by health care leadership and may act as a force to place quality improvement and patient safety at the top of an agenda.

OBSERVATION/ASSESSMENT/EVALUATION

This section of this article is the tactical portion where we discuss how to make a business case using a case-based vignette from a hospital known to the authors.

This tertiary-care free-standing children's hospital has a ten-bed pediatric intensive care unit (PICU) with an average census of eight patients. The hospital has recently embarked on initiatives targeted towards employee and staff safety (ESS). The hospital is self-insured for their employees, meaning any time an employee is off-work due to an occupational injury the organization pays for this from their finances. The hospital quality improvement team has over-exertion injuries (usually from lifting or pulling) as a component of their overall key-driver diagram to improve their ESS rate (injuries per hours worked).

The vignette above is very different than the clinical vignettes that we, as physicians, are used to reading in our literature. Note the points highlighting a service line and its growth, how employee injuries are paid, and the introduction of a novel quality improvement initiative on employee/staff safety.

The charge nurse has recently admitted a morbidly obese patient that requires almost a dozen staff members to help move each time a skin check, etc. is needed. This is dangerous as it pulls these employees away from their patients and importantly, the employees can hurt themselves with an over-exertion injury. The charge nurse's worst fear occurs one afternoon during a roll-over of the patient—a recent graduate from nursing school, pulls out his back. He immediately falls to the floor and is taken to the hospital's emergency department. He is out of work for two weeks and then returns on light-duty. The charge nurse wishes his unit had lifts to help move similar patients.

As we consider the charge nurse's goal to develop a compelling argument to convince the hospital to invest in lifts for his unit, we consider the components of an effective business case. There exist tremendous free on-line resources for constructing a business case that can walk a novice through the steps and outlines. A business case is an argument for an investment that contextualizes the costs for that investment with its projected financial benefits. These financial analyses usually point to increase in revenue (increase in number of customers or increase in pricing), cost reduction, or balance sheet improvements. In health care, the patients are the customers; at the same time, insurance companies and the government are also customers, because they are paying most of the operational revenue hospitals receive. Because quality and safety programs are usually not revenue generating, the financial analyses in business cases focus on cost reduction and other intangible benefits. Metrics like ROI that reflect the value quality and safety bring are effective financial tools.

In this vignette, the leader (charge nurse) is aware of the organizational work on Employee Staff Safety that the hospital has embarked on. The realm of employee and staff safety has started to gain momentum in the past few years. Like organization described in the vignette, many hospital systems are self-insured; they pay premiums to captive insurance companies, which are owned by the organization but are used to purchase reinsurance in which savings on the premiums can flow back to the parent organization. As such, health care managers and leaders can make a business case for investing in employee and staff safety programs, which generate cost savings that flow back to the organization.

For example, it may cost $25,000 to purchase a lift in the intensive care unit for morbidly obese patients. However, if the organization is going to embark on a bariatric surgery program, a business case is obvious: 1 employee overexertion (back injury) from not using a lift can result in the employee being out of work for 14 days ($35/h × 8 hours × 14 days = $3920). If we can demonstrate using the lift will save approximately 6 employees from an overexertion injury during the life of the product, then a business case can easily be constructed. There are complex assumptions that can be included, such as capitalization of the purchase, depreciation of the asset, the incremental increased annual salary. However, the point of this vignette is to show how simply a business case can begin to be developed for a quality improvement initiative. Beyond this singular story, organizations like Solutions for Patient Safety have incorporated this financial approach to provide "value calculators" for hospitals to calculate cost savings associated with quality and safety interventions that reduce hospital-acquired conditions based on actual historical data.[5]

Powerful business cases also include this financial data in the context of a compelling story. In health care, these are often subjective patient stories. For example, a patient with a preventable CLABSI that now must undergo additional procedures, prolong their hospital stay, and receive a long antibiotic course is 1 patient too many. Patient stories provide a burning platform for improvement, thereby making the financial argument more compelling.

GOALS

The goal of a leader is to ensure that their quality and safety work is prioritized by the organization; suffice it to say, simply asking and pleading is not a strategy. A key-driver diagram (KDD) based on the Institute of Healthcare's Model for Improvement is an excellent manner to demonstrate organizational alignment and commitment. The KDD contains a global aim that is at the 30,000-foot level that can be appreciated by senior leadership and the Board of Directors. A "global aim" for safety might be an absolute reduction in the rate of serious safety events. This goal then cascades to the level of a specific aim, which the respective KDD will be based on. A KDD is not the place to put in the dollars and make a financial case. In a formal presentation, after the global aim and KDD are shown, it may be prudent to show how attainment will result in a financial case and connect the dots between the global aim and specific financial achievements. The goal of the manager or leader is to have her work supported by making a continued business case for the work that distinctly ties back to the global aim. For example, if we know a hospital-acquired condition (eg, tracheostomy dislodgement) costs the organization approximately $5000 for each occurrence, then a pro forma (a manner to present financial projections over a time period) demonstrating an absolute reduction from 20 cases per year to 5 cases per year can quickly show a ROI of $75,000 (20 − 5 = 15; 15 × $5000).

DISCUSSION

As health care leaders, we must bridge the gap between frontline providers and Board members who make financial decisions. Using the previously discussed tactics to point out the direct cost benefits (money saved from decreasing hospital-acquired conditions, payments from insurance, keeping employees safe and therefore at work), one can advocate for the business case of quality improvement and patient/staff safety. Shifting the emphasis from a purely revenue-driven one to a more sustainable, long-term focus via quality improvement is the way of the future. Berwick[6] calls this moral change the "Era 3 of Medicine" and highlights improvement science as the way for health care organizations to attain success.

We have discussed the multitude of ways that quality improvement can offer cost benefits to a health care organization. One important point to add to this discussion reverts back to the original principle we learn as providers: to first do no harm. As technology and science continue to improve and contribute new ways to treat our patients, clinicians must continue to preserve their efforts to reduce harm when providing care. Combining the 2 ideals that we should always act to first do no harm and that there is a cost benefit to delivering safe health care, we can say simply that "doing the right thing pays."

At our own institution at Children's National Hospital (CNH), there is a culture of safety and emphasis placed on quality improvement, led by our President and Chief Executive Officer, Dr Kurt Newman. His adamant belief that "doing the right thing pays" is exemplified by multiple initiatives in place at CNH. An interprofessional simulation program, funded by a grant, was created at CNH to improve education for providers around process improvement methods. Employee Staff Safety is also of the utmost importance, shown by a recent quality improvement project reducing the number of employee injuries and, therefore, days away from work.[7]

Focus on the safety and well-being of employees adds to the overall culture of provider well-being, an idea that has become increasingly important in the time of the COVID-19 pandemic. In fact, the well-known Triple Aim has been increased to a Quadruple Aim to focus on improving the mental health of health care professionals, linking this to increased health care organization performance.[8] These examples of quality improvement and patient safety projects can be generalized from other health care leaders in how to improve the delivery of safety and quality at their respective hospitals and improving the bottom line, at the same time!

Ultimately, the onus is on the health care leader to contextualize the benefits of quality and safety work using financial data and patient stories. This is the nature of the problem for health care organization managers and leaders: they need to deliver the highest possible quality of care in the safest manner while making their margins.

CONTROVERSIES

"Why do I need to waste the time and effort to show my project saves the hospital money?" This is a quote that we unfortunately often hear. There is a moral argument made by many individuals that quality and safety initiatives are simply the "right thing to do." This is undoubtedly accurate. However, it costs money to do anything, be it the right or the wrong thing. It may certainly be controversial or anathema in your organization to broach the concept of financial return or business case vis-a-vis quality and safety. This sentiment is misguided in that in certain venues it may be inappropriate (eg, when discussing an issue with a family, when teaching front-line nurses about new equipment). However, despite the perceived controversy of discussing finances and business with regards to quality and safety, the onus is on the manager or leader to find the right time, place, and audience for these discussions. This trite statement is not easy to operationalize.

As leaders, we often find ourselves in venues where it is controversial to discuss the ROI for a particular quality or safety initiative. There will always be controversy surrounding the right time and place to have the discussions regarding the return on investing in a specific initiative. For example, 1 organization had a morbidly obese patient (almost 400 kg) that required 14 staff to turn the patient safely. During the care of that patient, the administration was criticized for not having a lift in each of the intensive care rooms to move these morbidly obese patients (each lift costs approximately $10,000). The timing of where and when to have such a discussion is important and potentially controversial. We suggest the manager or leader have these discussions regarding the business case away from the bedside within the right organizational structure and committees to make the purchasing decision.

FUTURE DIRECTIONS

Health care is a business. There is no group of individuals more suited than clinicians (providers, nurses, and so forth) to lead in health care. As the business demands of running a department, microsystem, service line, and so forth evolve, the need for leaders to have financial acumen has never been stronger. It is compulsory for quality and safety initiatives to be based on strong financial projections and assumptions. In the future, the need for robust financial/business cases will only be more intense. When planning a project, managers and leaders should ensure they have the tools ready to demonstrate what is needed in a business case *before* embarking on the initiative. This lesson holds true for us in health care organizations and in our respective specialty organizations. It is important in future work to collect baseline financial data, consider setting up the pro forma and financial documents to either make or refute a business case before starting the work. It is not a stretch to consider that soon all quality and safety initiatives in health care organizations will need an individual with strong financial background on the multidisciplinary team.

SUMMARY

Efforts to improve the quality and safety of patient and employees in health care organizations have made tremendous strides and gained significant influence in the past couple of decades. What was deemed "the right thing to do" in the early 2000s is now the fabric of providing care. As such, quality and safety have evolved to necessitating a business case to support continued investments in this crucial work. To do this, leaders and managers must use financial tools based on objective data coupled with subjective storytelling to make a compelling business case. Leveraging quality improvement methodologies, such as a KDD with simple-to-understand and quantify global aims, will help move the initiative in the right direction. Top organizations continue to invest in quality and safety and have evolved to developing robust models to support continued growth of efforts focused to deliver the highest quality of care for patients and families. Not investing in quality and safety efforts is financially the wrong decision. The investment pays off. As such, it is incumbent upon managers and leaders to make the business case. Soon, all quality and safety initiatives in health care organizations will need an individual with strong financial background on the multidisciplinary team. This article serves as a primer to begin understanding how to make the business case for quality and safety initiatives.

REFERENCES

1. Institute of Medicine (US) Committee on Quality of Health Care in America. In: Kohn LT, Corrigan JM, Donaldson MS, editors. To err is human: building a safer health system. Washington (DC): National Academies Press (US); 2000.

2. World Health Assembly, 72. Global action on patient safety. World Health Organization; 2019. Available at: https://apps.who.int/gb/ebwha/pdf_files/WHA72/A72_R6-en.pdf. Accessed August 17, 2021.
3. Berwick DM, Cassel CK. The NAM and the quality of health care - inflecting a field. N Engl J Med 2020;383(6):505–8.
4. Hilliard MA, Sczudlo R, Scafidi L, et al. Our journey to zero: reducing serious safety events by over 70% through high-reliability techniques and workforce engagement. J Healthc Risk Manag 2012;32(2):4–18.
5. Terao M, Hoffman JM, Brilli RJ, et al. Accelerating improvement in children's healthcare through quality improvement collaboratives: a synthesis of recent efforts. Curr Treat Options Peds 2019;5:111–30.
6. Berwick DM. Era 3 for medicine and health care. JAMA 2016;315(13):1329–30.
7. Fink A, Merkeley K, Tolliver C, et al. Reducing employee injury rates with a hospital-wide employee safety program. Pediatr Qual Saf 2021;6(2):e387.
8. Bodenheimer T, Sinsky C. From triple to quadruple aim: care of the patient requires care of the provider. The Ann Fam Med 2014;12(6):573–6.

New Payment Models

The Medicare Access and CHIP Reauthorization Act of 2015, Merit-based Incentive Payment System, Advanced Alternative Payment Models, Bundling, Value-Based Care, Quadruple Aim, and Big Data: What Do They Mean for Otolaryngology?

Stephen P. Cragle, MD

KEYWORDS

- ACO • Accountable care organization • CIN • Clinically integrated network • MIPS
- MACRA • APM • Value

KEY POINTS

- CMS and private payers are moving away from volume-based reimbursement to value-based reimbursement, utilizing a number of new payment models.
- The Affordable Care Act ("Obamacare") authorized CMS to develop several innovative payment models including the Quality Payment Program (QPP) and Accountable Care Organizations (ACO).
- Most Otolaryngologists are required to participate in the Merit-Based Incentive Payment System if they do not participate in an advanced alternate payment model such as an ACO.
- "Big Data" allows organizations to use clinical, actuarial, financial and claims data to identify opportunities for cost savings, improved safely and clinical quality and reducing barriers to care at the level of individual patients as well as trends for the entire network.

INTRODUCTION

New payment models have proliferated over the past decade since the advent of the Affordable Care and Patient Protection Act (ACA). A confusing array of acronyms and unfamiliar terms obscure an evolving paradigm shift in health care financing. Primary

St. Cloud Ear, Nose & Throat Clinic, PA, 1528 Northway Drive, St. Cloud, MN 56303, USA
E-mail address: scragle@stcloudent.com
Twitter: @docsadvice (S.P.C.)

Otolaryngol Clin N Am 55 (2022) 115–124
https://doi.org/10.1016/j.otc.2021.07.009
0030-6665/22/© 2021 Elsevier Inc. All rights reserved.

oto.theclinics.com

care seems to be most affected by the changing payment landscape, but otolaryngologists would do well to pay attention to the alterations because they represent the future for all providers. As the saying goes, if you're not at the table, you're probably on the menu.

In the summer of 2015, I was invited by our local health system to represent our single specialty ENT private practice group at a series of meetings exploring the formation of a regional accountable care organization (ACO) and clinically integrated network (CIN). The health system organized and financed the process; a total of 15 smaller hospitals and medical clinics appointed representatives. A consultant ushered us through a series of presentations and discussions, and ultimately most participants became comfortable with the idea of collaborating. I confess I initially attended to see what sort of mischief the health system was up to, having watched them consolidate and purchase several former private practice surgical specialty groups. Conversations with representatives of other groups confirmed my suspicions that they were participating for the same reason.

The group discussed ways to organize the network that acknowledged the health system's financial stake without allowing any 1 institution unilateral control of the decision-making process. The health system was awarded 3 board seats and each participating hospital or clinic was given 1 seat. I was nominated to chair the board of directors, presumably owing to nonalignment with the health system. I participated as board chair from 2015 to 2020, when I requested to step down and remain a board member. The process of creating a value-based organization dedicated to the triple aim of improving the experience of care, improving the health of populations, and decreasing per capita costs of health care[1] was quite valuable in understanding the changing landscape of health care delivery and reimbursement across the nation. I hope to communicate some insights and observations on this process that have relevance for the otolaryngologist.

VALUE-BASED CARE

Fee-for-service transactions have taken place between physicians and their patients from antiquity. In recent decades, this traditional model has come under scrutiny chiefly for its focus on payment for volume. Critics point to an increased use of medical services without a clear benefit over lower cost or more conservative measures. Value-based health care is a paradigm shift for health care stakeholders to redefine the delivery and payment of health care services based on health outcomes per unit of cost. This concept was introduced in 2006 by Michael Porter and Elizabeth Olmsted Teisberg in their book *Redefining Health Care* published by the Harvard Business Review Press.[2] Value is defined by the "measured improvement in a person's health outcomes for the cost of achieving that improvement."[3] The value proposition is not opposed to fee-for-service health financing per se, nor is it synonymous with the "triple aim," although people tend to commingle the terms. The use of clinical practice guidelines, best practices, quality improvement efforts, and efficiency promoters can certainly bend the cost curve and promote value under a fee-for-service arrangement. Value is contingent on improvement in a person's health outcome, which is not synonymous with the triple aim's population focus or experience of care focus. Value-based health care was embraced by President Obama early in his first term, and in a speech given before the 2009 annual meeting of the American Medical Association, he outlined in broad terms the concept of value-based health care reform,[4] some of which came to legislative fruition in the ACA, which are discussed elsewhere in this article.

TRIPLE AIM AND QUADRUPLE AIM

The Institute for Healthcare Improvement was founded by Donald Berwick and others in 1991 to further the science of quality improvement in health care.[5] Initially focused on identifying best practices in health care, the group went on to develop innovative health care delivery solutions and offered grants for the implementation of these innovations. In 2008, Don Berwick, Tom Nolan, and John Whittington described the concept of the "triple aim"[6]:

> Improving the U.S. health care system requires simultaneous pursuit of three aims: improving the experience of care, improving the health of populations, and reducing per capita costs of health care. Preconditions for this include the enrollment of an identified population, a commitment to universality for its members, and the existence of an organization (an "integrator") that accepts responsibility for all three aims for that population. The integrator's role includes at least five components: partnership with individuals and families, redesign of primary care, population health management, financial management, and macro system integration.

In 2014, Thomas Bodenheimer and Christine Sinsky added a fourth element—improving the work life of health care providers, including clinicians and staff—to create the "quadruple aim,"[7] arguing that, in light of the evidence of widespread physician burnout, the well-being of the health care team is a prerequisite for accomplishing the patient-centered focus of the triple aim.

THE AFFORDABLE CARE ACT AND MEDICARE ACCESS AND CHIP REAUTHORIZATION ACT OF 2015

The ACA, the controversial and comprehensive health care reform law enacted in March 2010 (sometimes known as ACA, PPACA, or "Obamacare"), had 3 primary goals. The first was to make affordable health insurance available to more people. The law provided individuals and families with subsidies (premium tax credits) that decrease insurance costs for households with incomes between 100% and 400% of the federal poverty level. Second, it expanded the Medicaid program to cover all adults with an income of less than 138% of the federal poverty level, although 14 states have yet to expand their Medicaid programs. Third, it encouraged innovative health care delivery methods designed to lower the costs of health care generally. This third aim authorized the Centers for Medicare and Medicaid Services (CMS) to develop a number of innovative delivery and payment models through the CMS Innovation Center including the Quality Payment Program (QPP) and ACO models.

THE MEDICARE ACCESS AND CHIP REAUTHORIZATION ACT OF 2015 AND THE QUALITY PAYMENT PROGRAM

The Medicare Access and CHIP Reauthorization Act of 2015 (MACRA) ended the sustainable growth rate formula, a flawed Medicare budgeting formula begun in 2003, which yearly threatened significant cuts in payments for participating Medicare providers, and required amendment yearly by congressional action. In addition to ending the sustainable growth rate, MACRA required the CMS to implement an incentive program, the QPP. Providers participating in Medicare Part B reimbursement were given 2 options to participate in the QPP: the Merit-based Incentive Payment System (MIPS) and Advanced Alternative Payment Models (APMs).[8] QPP started on January 1, 2017. Regardless of which program a clinician participates in, providers are evaluated on 4 core components: meaningful use of information technology, clinical quality, resource use (cost), and clinical practice improvement.[9] MACRA and the QPP (as discussed elsewhere in this article) are distinct from the ACA proper and remain the law even if all or part of the ACA is rescinded by legal action.[10]

THE MERIT-BASED INCENTIVE PAYMENT SYSTEM

The MIPS is a pay-for-performance system similar to a fee-for-service system, but adjusts future payments up or down based on prior care and physician comparison, either with peers in the same specialty or with themselves year over year. MIPS is the default QPP participation pathway for most otolaryngologists, although some private practice and academic groups or employed physicians work with institutions participating in an advanced APM.

MIPS is composed of 4 performance categories, which contribute a specified weight to the overall MIPS final score. For 2021 the categories are weighted as follows[11]:

- Quality: 30%
- Improvement activities: 15%
- Promoting interoperability: 25%
- Cost: 30%

CMS assigns a MIPS final score to individual clinicians, group practices, virtual groups, and APM entities. The final score reflects performance across the 4 categories and can range from 0 to 100 points. Participants can receive positive, neutral, or negative payment adjustments for every billed service for the payment year based on their final score from 2 years prior. The program was phased in over several years with increasing adjustment percentages, culminating in full vesting in 2020, which means a maximum adjustment of +9% or –9% for future years. The maximum adjustment was ±7% for 2019 reporting year. Based on final score comparisons between all participants, the 2019 final score correlated to 2021 payment adjustment as follows:

2019 Final Score	2021 Payment Adjustment
0–7.5 points	Negative MIPS payment adjustment of −7%
7.51–29.99 points	Negative MIPS payment adjustment, between 0% and 7%, on a linear sliding scale
30.00 points (performance threshold = 30.00 points)	Neutral MIPS payment adjustment (0%)
30.01–74.99 points	Positive (+) MIPS payment adjustment, >0%, on a linear sliding scale and multiplied by a scaling factor to preserve budget neutrality, not eligible for an additional adjustment for exceptional performance
75.00–100.00 points (additional performance threshold = 75.00 points)	Positive (+) MIPS payment adjustment, >0%, on a linear sliding scale and multiplied by a scaling factor to preserve budget neutrality and Additional positive (+) adjustment for exceptional performance on a linear sliding scale and multiplied by a scaling factor to proportionately distribute funds

In 2021, participants will need to score a total of at least 60 points to avoid a payment penalty in 2023. If an individual or group meets the requirements to report

MIPS and chooses not to in 2021, they will receive the full −9% Medicare payment adjustment in 2023. Participation is required in MIPS (unless otherwise exempt) if, in both 12-month segments of the MIPS determination period, you bill more than $90,000 for Part B covered professional services, see more than 200 Part B patients, and provide 200 or more covered professional services to Part B patients.

In addition to proper preparation, the assistance of a Qualified Clinical Data Registry is often required for medical clinics to meet their reporting requirements. A Qualified Clinical Data Registry is a CMS-approved entity that collects clinical data from MIPS clinicians and submits it to CMS on their behalf for MIPS reporting. MACRA has the power to negatively affect medical practices of all sizes in terms of progression, reimbursement, and advancement if reporting is incorrect or inaccurate. Two percent of all MIPS-eligible providers did not report in 2019, although most were covered by the MIPS Extreme and Uncontrollable Circumstances policy, which assigned these individual clinicians a neutral adjustment instead of the maximum negative payment adjustment.

MIPS payment adjustments are required by law to be budget neutral, which means that the projected positive payment adjustments must be balanced by the projected negative payment adjustments. As a result, MIPS-eligible clinicians with a 2019 final score between 30.01 and 74.99 points (22% of participants) will see a 2021 payment adjustment of 0.00%. Clinicians with a 2019 final score more than 75.00 points (74% of participants) will receive a positive adjustment ranging from 0.09% to a maximum of 1.79%. As a comparison, 96% of providers participating in a qualifying APM had MIPS scores at or greater than 75 points, giving virtually all of them a significant positive adjustment. Additionally, most of the latter group received a separate 5% bonus on all Part B payments as an additional benefit of advanced APM participation.[12]

ADVANCED ALTERNATE PAYMENT MODELS

APMs offer providers and hospitals greater flexibility and provide the highest reimbursement, although this comes with some risks. If a provider has the opportunity to take part in an advanced APM, they could earn a Medicare incentive payment for sufficiently participating in an innovative payment model.[13] If a provider or group sufficiently participate in an APM, they achieve qualifying APM participant, status which excludes them from MIPS participation and makes them eligible for a 5% APM incentive payment as noted elsewhere in this article.[14] A qualifying APM:

- Requires participants to use certified electronic health record technology;
- Provides payment for covered professional services based on quality measures comparable to those used in the MIPS quality performance category; and
- Either: (1) is a medical home model expanded under CMS Innovation Center authority OR (2) requires participants to bear a significant financial risk.

There are many APMs organized by the CMS Innovation Center covering disease-specific episodes and limited demographic groups, but the vast majority of providers participate in ACOs enrolled in the Medicare Shared Savings Program (MSSP).

ACCOUNTABLE CARE ORGANIZATIONS AND THE MEDICARE SHARED SAVINGS PROGRAM

The MSSP, introduced in 2012,[15] allows providers and hospitals to form an ACO to accept responsibility for the quality, cost, and experience of care (triple aim) of an assigned Medicare fee-for-service beneficiary population in exchange for an opportunity to share up to one-half of all savings on Medicare payments for the population.

This process represents a significant change along the continuum from volume toward value and outcomes. At-risk organizations need to optimize care coordination, manage risk corridors, decrease readmission rates, encourage alternatives to emergency room visits, increase the use of home health over skilled nursing facilities, and personalize care for high-spend outliers to lower their per capita spend below the benchmark set by CMS. Quality benchmarks ensure that the savings is not achieved solely by decreasing access to care. Enhanced risk and reward set this program apart from MIPS and other pay-for-performance programs:

- Risk: most MSSP ACOs bear at least some downside risk: if the ACO spend exceeds the CMS-determined benchmark for the specified population beyond a preselected risk corridor, the ACO will pay CMS one-half of the excess spend.
- Reward: MSSP ACOs receive up to 50% of all shared savings generated by spending less per capita than the benchmark set by CMS. The full share is only available if all quality benchmarks were also reached. In addition, all participating providers receive a 5% bonus to all their part B payments as a consequence of participating in an advanced APM.[16]

Eligible ACOs may also apply for a skilled nursing facility 3-day rule waiver to facilitate decreases in inpatient stays for patients who need skilled nursing care and may establish and operate a beneficiary incentive program and use expanded telehealth services. Many ACOs use data mining services that can identify beneficiaries with higher than expected expenses to allow optimized care coordination to decrease their spend. These services can also identify providers with cost and/or quality data that significantly lag benchmarks and can trigger quality improvement measures or even dismissal from the ACO.

Currently, 477 ACOs cover 10.7 million Medicare beneficiaries, about 25% of all Medicare beneficiaries. Most ACOs are in metropolitan areas, but some rural areas have found success in the Shared Savings Program. MSSP ACOs vary in the relative participation by primary care and specialist physicians, but the opportunities for realizing savings invite efforts by both groups. Although financial pressures and economies of scale have led to consolidation (such as health systems purchasing or competing with physician private practices), it is not clear that tight integration is necessary for optimal results as ACOs of varying integration have all produced modest improvements in cost and quality.[15]

CLINICALLY INTEGRATED NETWORKS

CINs are similar to ACOs, but are separate legal entities. ACUs could be thought of as a subset of CINs strictly for Medicare beneficiaries. In August 1996, the US Department of Justice and the Federal Trade Commission released joint "Statements of Antitrust Enforcement Policy in Health Care,"[17] which addressed physician–hospital organizations and other groups' desire to integrate clinically to streamline care and facilitate favorable insurance contract negotiation. This guideline formed the legal basis to form CINs involving independent hospitals and provider groups, and covered safe harbor guidelines, basic requirements, and economic and clinical integration pathways. The widespread adoption of CINs did not take place for a number of years, but in the past decade or so many hospitals and provider groups have formed CINs:

Health systems are using CINs to adapt to competitive environments and changing payment policies in several ways. CINs allow health systems to (1) move care into lower-cost settings while retaining referral pathways for their tertiary facilities; (2) extend their geographic reach without the capital and administrative costs of

*acquiring and onboarding; (3) maximize negotiating leverage while reducing con-
tracting burden; and (4) offer advantages (such as electronic health record and
quality reporting support) to physicians while allowing them to remain in independent practice.*[18]

CINs have much more flexibility regarding the form of integration and the extent of
cooperation between integrated organizations than do ACOs and generally extend to
private payers. Many such agreements can lead to participation in bundling for specific service lines such as total joint episode payments and even full capitation for
defined populations of insureds. Some CINs have been configured to create so-
called narrow networks that may create competition among specialty groups vying
to join the CIN to avoid losing a large number of referrals from participating primary
care providers. Some well-established networks give scorecards to providers
comparing them with their peers within the network regarding cost and quality benchmarks, and outliers with higher spend and/or lower quality scores may be dismissed
from the network. These mature CINs often seek full risk for some of their service lines,
with capitation via per patient per month, especially for primary care. Most specialists
continue to be paid by discounted fee-for-service arrangement, and specialty costs
tend to be decreased by efforts to decrease specialist consultations.

BUNDLING

The CMS Innovation Center has numerous bundled payment models covering specific
populations of beneficiaries such as:

- Comprehensive Care for Joint Replacement Model
- Comprehensive ESRD (End Stage Renal Disease) Care Model
- Oncology Care Model
- Bundled Payments for Care Improvement Advanced Model

All of these programs are themselves advanced APMs involving specific episodes of
care where clinicians accept some risk for their patients' quality and cost outcomes
and meet other specified criteria.

As mentioned elsewhere in this article, CINs often seek bundled contracts for specific episodes of care such as total joints, oncology, and end-stage renal disease. In
addition, some practices seek bundled payments directly with payers and hospitals
or ambulatory surgical centers to decrease global costs to the payer while incentivizing providers to decrease costs and improve quality. The hospital or ASC together
with the physician group receive a fixed payment for the entire episode of care. If costs
are higher than the expected benchmarks, the group realizes less payment, and if
costs are lower, there is more for the providers and hospital or ASC to share.

BIG DATA

This ambiguous term represents various efforts by value-oriented organizations to use
patient, provider, and organizational data for analysis. This work usually includes
claims data, clinical data, actuarial data, and financial data to provide comprehensive
and often very granular information for retrospective and sometimes even real-time
analysis. By mining large repositories of data and correlating often disparate and
seemingly unrelated streams, very specific processes can be created to identify financial and clinical trends, recognize outliers among patients, providers, and systems,
and create novel solutions that promote value. Qualified clinical data registries represent one such effort, although many health systems, insurance plans, and CMS itself

also carry out a similar data analysis. This process can drive innovation, safety, and cost reductions for health care, thus driving the value proposition.

IMPLICATIONS FOR OTOLARYNGOLOGISTS

Many otolaryngologists will continue to report quality and cost data to CMS via the MIPS program. A small positive payment adjustment is possible for high-performing practices. It may be prudent to use a Qualified Clinical Data Registry such as the American Academy of Otolaryngology–Head and Neck Surgery's Reg-ent registry to streamline and strengthen MIPS reporting. A specialty-specific registry like Reg-ent has the added ability to define and develop specialty-specific quality measures and define the value of otolaryngology services for future iterations of public and private value-based payment models.[19]

ACOs have the potential to advance the triple aim, but it may come at the cost of consolidation and inappropriate risk for providers.[20] Many health systems continue to see benefits in starting their own specialist programs or purchasing private practice specialty groups. Otolaryngologists in solo practice, small single specialty groups, and multispecialty groups not aligned with a health system would do well to examine opportunities to participate in an ACO for several reasons. First, otolaryngologists who have the opportunity to participate in an MSSP ACO could see payments in the form of shared savings, although payment is usually tied to attribution, which usually favors primary care physicians over specialists. Conversely, the same focus on primary care would shield a specialist to some degree against a payback situation should the ACO fail to produce expected shared savings. Second, ACO staff generally report quality and cost data on behalf of all participating providers, which usually exempts the otolaryngologist from MIPS reporting. Finally, participating in an advanced APM (MSSP ACOs generally qualify) entitles the provider to a 5% bonus on all part B payments for that year. This bonus sunsets in 2024 and will be replaced by a yearly fee schedule update of 0.75% (vs non-APM participants' 0.25%) starting in 2026.[21]

Otolaryngologist participation in CINs and bundling programs should be considered individually given local factors such as degree of integration, competition for referrals, and availability of partnerships with hospitals, ASCs, and willing payers. Health systems and payers are increasingly looking for predictability in health care spending, and many look favorably on agreements that invite limited risk sharing by providers and create upside incentive for decreasing costs and improving safety. Be vigilant for narrow networks and other efforts to create competition for referrals, and consider the local market before signing network agreements. Full-risk capitation is unlikely for most specialists in CIN and bundling arrangements, but it pays to study one's practice for the kind of data that payers and health systems understand so that if full capitation contracts or bundles are offered, you can respond from a data-driven understanding of risks and rewards.

New payment models and value-based health care are the future of medicine. With an understanding of various models and the attendant risks and rewards, otolaryngologists can survive and even thrive in this new era.

CLINICS CARE POINTS

- Pay attention to your MIPS reporting process—opportunities do exist for positive payment adjustments, but the price for inaccuracy can be high.

- Consider using a Qualified Clinical Data Registry such as Reg-ent to streamline and improve MIPS reporting.
- Consider participating in a local/regional Accountable Care Organization and/or a Clinically Integrated Network; if you are not at the table, your practice or specialty may be on the menu!
- Be aware of opportunities to participate with payers and health systems in bundled procedures. Socrates' maxim "know thyself" applies here: a deep and first-hand understanding of your own practice will serve you well when it comes time to negotiate partial risk-sharing agreements.

DISCLOSURE

S.P. Cragle is a member and former chair, board of governors of Central Minnesota Health Network, an Accountable Care Organization and Clinically Integrated Network.

REFERENCES

1. The IHI triple aim. Available at: http://www.ihi.org/Engage/Initiatives/TripleAim/Pages/default.aspx. Accessed May 24, 2021.
2. Porter M, Teisberg E. Redefining health care. Boston (MA): Harvard Business Review Press; 2006.
3. Elizabeth T, Scott W, O'Hara S. Defining and implementing value-based health care: a strategic framework. Acad Med 2020;95(5):682–5.
4. Remarks by the president to the annual conference of the American Medical Association. Available at: https://obamawhitehouse.archives.gov/the-press-office/remarks-president-annual-conference-american-medical-association. Accessed May 24, 2021.
5. Institute for healthcare improvement. Available at: http://www.ihi.org/about/pages/history.aspx. Accessed May 24, 2021.
6. Berwick DM, Nolan TW, Whittington J. The triple aim: care, health, and cost. Health Aff 2008;27(3):759–69.
7. Bodenheimer T, Sinsky C. From triple to quadruple aim: care of the patient requires care of the provider. The Ann Fam Med 2014;12(6):573–6.
8. Quality payment program overview. Available at: https://qpp.cms.gov/about/qpp-overview. Accessed May 24, 2021.
9. MACRA in the era of big data: implications for clinical practice. Available at: https://doi.org/10.1016/j.ijcard.2018.02.080. Accessed May 24, 2021.
10. Affordable Care Act (ACA). Available at: https://www.healthcare.gov/glossary/affordable-care-act/. Accessed May 24, 2021.
11. 2021 Merit-based Incentive Payment System (MIPS) Payment Year Payment Adjustment Fact Sheet, CMS. Available at: https://qpp-cm-prod-content.s3.amazonaws.com/uploads/1110/2021%20MIPS%20Payment%20Adjustment%20Fact%20Sheet.pdf.
12. Quality payment program participation in 2019: results at-a-glance. Available at: https://qpp.cms.gov/resources/resource-library. Accessed May 24, 2021.
13. Quality payment program. Available at: https://www.cms.gov/Medicare/Quality-Payment-Program/Quality-Payment-Program. Accessed May 24, 2021.
14. How MIPS eligibility is determined. Available at: https://qpp.cms.gov/mips/how-eligibility-is-determined. Accessed May 24, 2021.

15. Fisher ES, Shortell SM, Kreindler SA, et al. A framework for evaluating the formation, implementation, and performance of accountable care organizations. Health Aff 2012;31(11):2368–78.
16. Advanced Alternate Payment Models (APMs). Available at: https://qpp.cms.gov/apms/advanced-apms. Accessed May 24, 2021.
17. Available at: https://www.justice.gov/atr/page/file/1197731/download. Accessed May 24, 2021.
18. Ridgely MS, Timbie J, Duffy E, et al. Consolidation by any other name? The emergence of clinically integrated networks. Health Serv Res 2020;55:114.
19. About Reg-entsm. Available at: https://www.entnet.org/about-reg-ent. Accessed May 24, 2021.
20. Colla CH, Fisher ES. Moving forward with accountable care organizations: some answers, more questions. JAMA Intern Med 2017;177(4):527–8.
21. MACRA frequently asked questions. Available at: https://www.aamc.org/what-we-do/mission-areas/health-care/macra/faq. Accessed May 24, 2021.

Marketing Your Practice
Setting Yourself Apart in a Competitive Market, Online Reputation Building, and Managing Patient Experience/Satisfaction

Leslie Kim, MD, MPH[a],*, Dale Amanda Tylor, MD, MPH[b],
Christopher Y. Chang, MD[c]

KEYWORDS

- Marketing • Branding • Physician branding • Online reputation • Patient experience
- Patient satisfaction • Online reviews

KEY POINTS

- In today's digital age, physicians need to understand how to compete in this new practice climate by successfully marketing online through an updated practice website and social media.
- Actively engaging in online personal branding as a physician can greatly influence how others perceive you and the value they give to your services as a surgeon.
- Optimizing patient satisfaction improves clinical outcomes, reimbursement, patient referrals, and retention. Unsatisfied patients may be effectively managed using the H.E.A.R.T. approach.

INTRODUCTION

In the past, there were far fewer options when it came to marketing a medical practice. Marketing was limited to print, referrals, and word of mouth. For patients, researching a physician practice was limited to recommendations by their friends and their own physicians. It was, therefore, much more difficult for patients to identify the best health care provider for their problem. It was also much more difficult for physicians to target potential patients in a meaningful way or calculate return on investment.

[a] Department of Otolaryngology–Head and Neck Surgery, The Ohio State University Wexner Medical Center, 915 Olentangy River Road, Suite 4000, Columbus, OH 43212, USA; [b] Riviera ENT, Cottage Hospital Santa Barbara, 1819 State Street, Suite A, Santa Barbara, CA 93101, USA; [c] Fauquier Ear, Nose, and Throat Consultants, 550 Hospital Drive, Warrenton, VA 20186, USA
* Corresponding author.
E-mail address: Leslie.Kim@osumc.edu
Twitter: @DrLeslieKim (L.K.); @rivieraentsb (D.A.T.); @FauquierENT (C.Y.C.)

Otolaryngol Clin N Am 55 (2022) 125–135
https://doi.org/10.1016/j.otc.2021.08.005
oto.theclinics.com

Now, things are different. It is no longer enough to publish your number in the Yellow Pages, take out an ad in the local newspaper, or send out some mailers and then wait for patients to come to you. Not only is the market more competitive but also patients now have more access to health information at their fingertips. People no longer exclusively obtain their news from newspapers[1] but turn to a plethora of digital resources to research their symptoms, their conditions, and their physicians.

It is commonplace now for prospective patients to investigate their doctors online[2] well in advance of their first visit. This means that physicians need to understand how to compete in this new practice climate by effectively promoting themselves.

SETTING YOURSELF APART IN A COMPETITIVE MARKET

As patients are increasingly turning to a vast array of online sources[3] for health care information, the digital marketplace has become a crowded space with a multitude of platforms and content. Patients are discovering health information (and misinformation) on search engines, blogs, websites, and social media sites such as Instagram, Snapchat, Facebook, YouTube, and more. It is estimated that there are over 1 billion searches for health-related content on Google[4] every single day. Many of these searches will be potential opportunities for prospective patients to find your practice.

Benefits of an Online Presence

Online information management can improve physician reputation and can bring more patients through a practice's doors, when compared to traditional offline marketing. Some other benefits include,

- Can be more cost-effective. Social media is considered free, other than the time spent creating and interacting on it. There are options to pay for targeted advertising.
- Easier to keep up-to-date. Rather than a lengthy design, review, and print process that can be expensive, time-consuming, and cumbersome to update, an online presence means you can share new information or developments at the touch of a button.
- More sustainable. Reduced print, paper, and recycling costs with an online presence.
- Face-to-face contact can be reduced. Although there is a lot to be said when it comes to in-person patient contact, some conversations, research, and discussions can take place online. Furthermore, health education obtained online can also make office visits more productive, especially if the information was obtained with materials that a medical practice has itself produced.
- Easier to target. Social media in particular makes targeting patients easy. Between hashtags, online searches, and targeted ads, a medical practice can reach patients with more precision than ever. Conversely, a wider reach can be obtained relative to printed marketing materials on this basis.
- Easier to track return on investment. With targeting, analytics, and exact results versus spending, you can really break down what marketing activity is working for you and your practice.
- Build a real-time feedback loop. With the increased focus on reviews[5] that comes with an online presence, a medical practice can get immediate feedback from patients allowing for immediate practice change implementations when and where necessary.

Reputation is no longer confined to professional circles and patients. Many other people including peers you have not met, prospective patients, and media professionals will get to know a practice online well before meeting any of a practice's physicians.

Challenges of Building an Online Presence

One of the biggest challenges for a physician trying to establish a robust online presence is HIPAA and patient confidentiality. How do you share specific, targeted content — image and video-based content at that — without breaching these guidelines?

Patient consent and anonymization is key. Private health information (PHI) should *never* be shared on social media. Even if it is the most interesting case you have ever seen, or you know that your social media audience will love it, you cannot share content that will reveal PHI in text, images, or video, without patient consent.

PHI being private is a well-understood and accepted concept. However, a study that analyzed patient information shared on the hashtag #ShareAStoryInOneTweet estimated that 32% of the stories shared by medical professionals[6] included information that could lead to a patient being identified by a friend or family member. In the same study, it was estimated that 46% of tweets could lead to a patient being able to recognize themselves.

It is also worth being aware of the possibility of negative feedback or harassment online. It is an unfortunate side effect of the digital age, but people tend to think less about an individual person at the end of a message they send. That being said, health care professionals should not avoid useful digital tools because of this risk. In fact, having an active and strong digital presence can actually help you to be in control of your own reputation.

Another challenge is keeping your online presence up-to-date with correct information, fresh content, and relevant information for your audience. As online information is constantly being updated and refreshed, it takes consistent time and effort to maintain your digital reputation. People expect to be able to find information about another person online and are increasingly interpreting a lack of online presence as negative.

There is also the question of whether to interact with commenters, questions, and messages online. Anything that could be construed as medical advice or responses to specific medical questions should be avoided. You may wish to respond to comments that are more generic in nature, especially to build engagement as you grow your presence online.

Online marketing takes time and effort. It is not an instant win unless a significant amount of time and even some money is invested, and even then, it is not a guarantee. The likelihood is that at first, your follower numbers and engagement will remain low. In the beginning, most traffic will solely come from patients visiting your website for more information. Indeed, it may take *years* for significant digital traffic to accumulate beyond this core patient traffic, even with consistent content production (**Figs. 1–3**), and you should not become discouraged with disappointing numbers, especially if you are starting out from scratch.

Active Versus Passive Marketing

In the end, the ultimate goal is for a patient visit to occur. All efforts online and offline should be geared toward this singular goal. Toward that end, all digital social media accounts and offline presences should work together collaboratively to drive traffic toward a medical practice's website. This synergy between online and offline presence can further build reputation and legitimacy in the eyes of potential patients.

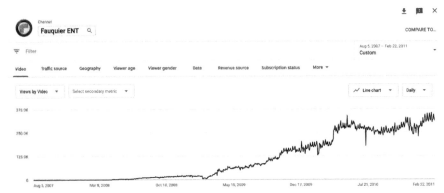

Fig. 1. YouTube traffic for Dr Christopher Chang. (*Courtesy of* Dr. Christopher Chang, MD, Warrenton, Virginia (youtube.com/fauquierent).)

Active versus passive marketing is also something to consider. *Active marketing* is a more upfront way where you broadcast your individual expertise and display it in a way that brings focus to you and your business. It is deliberate, purposeful, and requires effort to tell people why you are the health care professional for them, why they should call you for an appointment, and why you are absolutely the best at what you do. It can feel a little like a hard sell and can turn some patients off although others love it.

Passive marketing is more of an approach where you provide information, guidance, and expertise but let patients make their own decisions on what they do next. It has less of a focus on the individual physician or practice and more of an "if you build it, they will come" ethos. Neither approach is right or wrong, but it is something to consider as you build and grow your online presence. Authenticity is the key thing to create, whether as an active or passive marketer.

Do not forget to regularly measure how you are doing by using robust analytics and checking your statistics frequently. This allows you to see what is working and what is not and then to respond accordingly to optimize further growth.

ONLINE REPUTATION BUILDING
Personal Brand Versus Personal Branding

Whether we like it or not, each of us has a *personal brand*. And your personal brand is your reputation; it is how others view your expertise, personality, values, and

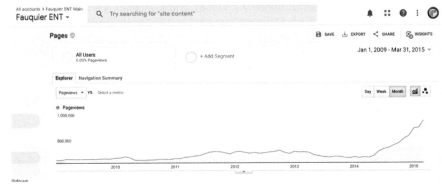

Fig. 2. Practice website traffic for Dr Christopher Chang (fauquierent.net). (*Courtesy of* Dr. Christopher Chang, MD, Warrenton, Virginia (youtube.com/fauquierent).)

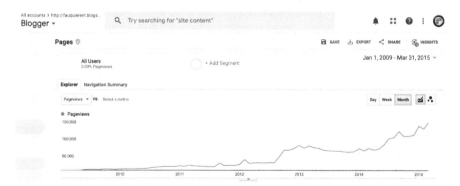

Fig. 3. Blog traffic for Dr Christopher chang (blog.fauquierent.net). (*Courtesy of* Dr. Christopher Chang, MD, Warrenton, Virginia (blog.fauquierent.net).)

mission—what others are thinking or saying about you. This is not to be confused with *personal branding*, which is the strategy used to help build your personal brand—what you are saying about yourself.

The idea of personal branding makes many people, and especially physicians, uncomfortable. But the reality is, in today's digital world, if you do not take control of your personal brand both online and off-line, then you are not only missing out on opportunities but also permitting others to control your narrative.

While you cannot completely control your personal brand (such as what others are saying about you), you can certainly try by actively engaging in personal branding: By purposefully communicating who you are, you can greatly influence how others perceive you and the value they give to your services as a surgeon.[7]

Google Yourself

Seventy-seven percent of adults start looking for health information online on a search engine,[8] so it is prudent to Google yourself and see what this brings up. Most users only view the first page (first ten website links) of Google search results,[9] so the information provided on the first page can highly impact your online reputation and personal brand as a physician.

Unfortunately, most physicians have little to no control over the content that patients and potential patients discover on that first page. This is because for most, the first page of Google search results is dominated by commercially controlled, third-party physician information and rating websites such as Healthgrades and Vitals.[10] For nearly half of otolaryngologists, a ratings website appeared higher on a Google search than their own professional website.[11] As a result, many of us are put in a situation where public opinion is more readily available than physician-curated content.

Physician Rating Websites

When making decisions about health care, people often rely on the advice of others. Physician rating websites (PRWs) such as Healthgrades and Vitals are online platforms where users can check physicians' profiles, ratings, and reviews, in their search for a suitable physician.

Several studies show that most ratings and reviews posted on PRWs are fortunately positive. However, negative comments and ratings can certainly have a direct negative influence on a person's decision to visit a physician.[12]

Factors that have been shown in several studies to be associated with higher ratings on PRWs include younger age, fewer years in practice, increased online presence, and greater number of reviews.[12,13] The potentially modifiable factors are the latter two.

Increased online presence is often seen in younger or less experienced physicians who are more likely to use social media and online marketing than their older or more experienced counterparts. Additionally, PRWs are more popular with younger patients,[14] who may have a better personal connection with physicians of a similar age, leading to higher ratings.[15]

What also matters is the number of user reviews. The sheer number of recommendations that a physician has on his/her profile can influence a user's decisions on whether to visit the physician or not. In other words, users of PRWs are more likely to visit physicians who are positively reviewed by a large number of users.[13]

As physicians, we have very limited control over the information that ultimately gets published on these rating sites. However, one potential strategy is to proactively ask happy patients to leave reviews on these sites (Healthgrades generally occupies a higher rank on Google search results than Vitals) in an effort to not only increase the number of positive user reviews but also dilute out the negative ones as well.

Another way to mitigate negative online reviews goes back to increasing online presence. Physician social media usage has been shown to decrease the Google search position of negative online reviews,[16] and active social media profiles can displace third-party rating websites from appearing on the top of physician Google search results altogether.[17]

The Role of Social Media

In training, you are taught that if you take great care of patients and perform good surgery, then patients will come. While there is truth to this, the traditional methods of practice building such as surgeon pedigree, referrals, and word of mouth are becoming increasingly supplanted by a new paradigm based on social media presence.

Social media is somewhat redefining the concept of physician expertise and online reputation to the lay public. One study found that while the total number of social media followers was associated with Google front page placement for "top 20 plastic surgeons," medical school ranking and years in practice were not.[18]

Patients gravitate online toward surgeons with influence, and that influence is increasingly being defined by (whether we like it or not) likes and followers. And this effect is exponential; the more likes and followers you have, the more easily you will obtain more likes and followers. You can therefore achieve perceived expertise through your social media presence, regardless of your experience.

Social media is a powerful tool for personal branding as a physician. The content that you put out on social media platforms such as Facebook, Instagram, YouTube, Twitter, LinkedIn, Snapchat, and TikTok is fully yours. And this self-curated content can displace third-party rating sites, improve front page Google placement, and most importantly, allow better control of your online reputation.

Pearls and Pitfalls of Online Reputation Building

- Define your purpose. Identify the qualities about you (your expertise, personality, values, and goals) as a physician that you want to showcase online. Then Google yourself to see how your online reputation or personal brand *today* aligns with your purpose.

- Strategize how you want to deliver your content. Assess your strengths to determine how you want to deliver content to your target audience (text, photos, videos, voice, and so forth).
- Get on social media. Start by picking a handle (consider using your name and degree, the crux of your personal brand) and try to own it across all platforms, even ones you do not think you will use. Be thoughtful about your bio. Be consistent in posting valuable content and engage with others in your target audience to grow a following.
- Be authentic without compromising on professionalism. The internet is forever. Before posting anything, ask yourself: "Would my family and friends be okay with it? My boss and work colleagues? My patients?" Check institutional regulations and policies where applicable, and of course, no HIPAA violations.
- Be proactive about online reviews. Ask happy patients to write online reviews (Google, Healthgrades, Vitals, and so forth) to not only improve your online rating (the more positive reviews the better) but also dilute out any negative reviews as well.

MANAGING PATIENT EXPERIENCE/SATISFACTION
Patient Experience Versus Patient Satisfaction

Patient experience and patient satisfaction are often used in an interchangeable fashion, but these terms are not equivalent. *Patient experience* involves the interactions between the patient and a given health care practice or system, including care provided by physicians, nurses, and ancillary staff; the facility; and coordination with insurance plans. It encompasses access to appointments, health information, and communication tools. Respect for patient needs, values, and preferences is included.

With *patient satisfaction,* the important consideration is if the patient's expectations of the delivery of their health care have been met. It is an indicator of how well a patient is being treated in a medical practice, from standpoints of quality of care and from how happy the patient is with the care provided.[19] Expectations can vary considerably between individual patients, which can result in very different perceptions in satisfaction despite patients receiving similar care for similar health problems.[20]

The Price of Patient Satisfaction

The Institute of Medicine, in their influential 2001 "Crossing the Quality Chasm" report, included six aims for the health care system focusing on safe, effective, patient-centered, timely, efficient, and equitable care.[21] The Centers for Medicare and Medicaid Services, with the passage of the Patient Protection and Affordable Care Act in 2010, has linked physician and hospital reimbursement to patient satisfaction. The problem with this valuation of patient satisfaction is that higher patient satisfaction in the inpatient setting is associated with higher health care utilization, more inpatient care, greater use of prescription drugs, and a corresponding increased mortality rate.[22]

The importance that patient satisfaction surveys have been given by payers and employers and the public has led to considerable negative impact among physicians, and this may be a source of burnout. Indeed, in one study among American otolaryngologists, 63.8% found that the monitoring did not result in a positive impact to their practice, and 36.2% believed it resulted in pressure to order unnecessary diagnostic testing or inappropriate prescriptions.[23] Unfortunately, the reality is that clinicians today need to embrace patient satisfaction to succeed in clinical practice.

Elements of Patient Satisfaction

In many cases, the elements of satisfaction mirror the elements of patient-centered care.

Picker.org has identified 8 principles of person-centered care that can be applied to provide consistent care of high quality[24]:

- Fast access to reliable health care advice
- Effective treatment delivered by trusted professionals
- Continuity of care and smooth transitions
- Involvement and support for family and caregivers
- Clear information, communication, and support for self-care
- Involvement in decisions and respect for preferences
- Emotional support, empathy, and respect
- Attention to physical and environmental needs

Although we may not be able to address all these factors with each patient encounter, being cognizant of them can lead to an improved patient experience and, by extension, improved patient satisfaction.

Benefits of Optimizing Patient Satisfaction

There are several reasons why a practice would want to value patient satisfaction[25]:

- Improved clinical outcomes. Patients with higher trust in their health care provider report less symptoms,[26] greater satisfaction with treatment, higher quality of life, and better health behaviors, although it should be reinforced that some outcomes are worse in satisfied patients whose providers may be acquiescing to unnecessary studies and treatments.
- Improved reimbursement. Higher patient satisfaction scores can translate into increased patient volume and additional revenue; conversely, lower patient satisfaction scores are associated with a loss of patient volume and loss of revenue. Providers may charge more for their services if they have excellent patient satisfaction scores without decreasing market share or profit. There is also an inverse correlation between patient satisfaction rates and costly medical malpractice suits.
- Improved patient referrals and retention. Satisfied patients will share their positive experience with others just as unsatisfied patients will share their negative experiences. A positive digital presence will not only attract patients to you but will help prevent establish patients from seeking care elsewhere.

Ways to Improve Patient Satisfaction

Some methods to maximize patient satisfaction and retention are as follows[27]:

- Create and foster an online presence to showcase your brand
- Offer online scheduling and communication
- Provide appointment confirmations and reminders
- Have clinical forms available online to streamline intake
- Be friendly: Clinical and nonclinical staff should all project helpful and positive attitudes at all times, from check-in to check-out
- Ensure inviting, clean, and comfortable facilities
- Minimize wait times where possible
- Spend adequate time with patients; bedside manner counts

- Survey patients after appointments to gauge strengths and areas in need of improvement
- Respond to online feedback promptly

Managing Unsatisfied Patients

In business, the concept of *service recovery* involves the process of restoring customer confidence after a service breakdown occurs. Applying this to medicine means having a strategy in place so that unsatisfied patients feel that their concerns are heard and responded to. All members of the health care team must be engaged to quickly turn a problematic experience into a positive one for a patient.

H.E.A.R.T. is an acronym that is well-suited to addressing patient complaints:

- *Hear.* Allow the patient to talk or vent without interruption. This is a crucial first step. Show compassion with positive body language. Ask questions to clarify any assumptions. This sets the stage for an unsatisfied patient to become more open to solutions your practice offers.
- *Empathize.* Name the patient's emotion, such as frustration or anger, and then validate it as understandable. This helps the patient know that you are trying to understand their perspective and are treating them with respect.
- *Apologize.* A sincere apology for a negative experience can be powerful. This is not an admission of guilt but rather demonstration that you and your practice cares. Avoid shifting blame or becoming defensive.
- *Respond.* Many complaints stem from unmet expectations. Re-establish a new expectation by providing a list of possible options to resolve the problem. Your response should be as immediate as possible, or they should be provided with a timeframe to expect the response.
- *Thank.* Thank the patient for the chance to correct their problem. This solidifies for them that their concerns were valid, addressed, and that they have helped you to improve your process.

Addressing Negative Online Reviews

When dealing with online patient reviews, there is more emotion and more risk involved. Such reviews can be seen by a wide audience of prospective patients and can cloud what other patients perceive of the care you provide, regardless of their basis in fact. Responding to online reviews can be dangerous if violation of patient privacy laws occurs or if the response is viewed as combative or negative.

There is some general guidance on what to do and not to do in responding to bad online reviews[28,29]:

What to do:

- If feasible, respond first offline, by phone or in person, to discuss their concerns. Use the H.E.A.R.T. method mentioned previously. It is possible that this personal contact may lead to the patient revising or removing the review.
- Only respond with general protocols/policies instead of specifically mentioning the reviewer. For example, state that each patient is thoroughly assessed for a given concern and that treatment depends on a patient's individual situation.
- Ensure that your online profile is professional and current on your own website, on search engines, and on health rating websites.
- Remember that most reviews are good, and one bad review may not be as destructive as it feels it will be. Proactively increase your number of positive online reviews by soliciting feedback from happy patients.

- Focus on the reviews found on the most trafficked websites (Google, Healthgrades, Vitals, and so forth).with the largest audiences.
- Be proactive in asking all patients about their experiences up front so that you can hone your office's process of optimizing patient satisfaction.

What not to do:

- Do not immediately respond online to negative reviews. Take time to compose your thoughts to prevent them from seeming angry, threatening, or petty. Never threaten litigation in a public fashion.
- Never disclose that the patient has a relationship with your practice or that they were ever in your office. It is against HIPAA to do so without a patient's expressed permission, and even their review is not considered consent to release anything related to their care.
- Do not hide from online reviews as they are a reality of patient care today.

DISCLOSURE

The authors have nothing to disclose.

REFERENCES

1. Shearer E. Social media outpaces print newspapers in the U.S. as a news source. 2018. Available at: https://www.pewresearch.org/fact-tank/2018/12/10/social-media-outpaces-print-newspapers-in-the-u-s-as-a-news-source/. Accessed August 1, 2021.
2. Sharon Swee-Lin T, Goonawardene N. Internet health information seeking and the patient-physician relationship: a systematic review. J Med Internet Res 2017; 19(1):e9.
3. Chen Y, et al. Health information obtained from the internet and changes in medical decision making: questionnaire development and cross-sectional survey. J Med Internet Res 2018;20(2):e47.
4. Drees J. Google receives more than 1 billion health questions every day. 2019. Available at: https://www.beckershospitalreview.com/healthcare-information-technology/google-receives-more-than-1-billion-health-questions-every-day.html. Accessed August 1, 2021.
5. Hong YA, et al. What do patients say about doctors online? A systematic review of studies on patient online reviews. J Med Internet Res 2019;21(4):e12521.
6. Ahmed W, et al. Public disclosure on social media of identifiable patient information by health professionals: content analysis of twitter data. J Med Internet Res 2020;22(9):e19746.
7. Crowe C. Essential marketing tips: build your own brand one step at a time. Facial Plast Surg Clin N Am 2010;18:499–502.
8. Majority of adults look online for health information. Pew Research Center. Available at: https://www.pewresearch.org/fact-tank/2013/02/01/majority-of-adults-look-online-for-health-information. Accessed June 2, 2021.
9. Sharp E. The first page of Google, by the numbers. ProtoFuse; 2014. Available at: www.protofuse.com/blog/first- page-of-google-by-the-numbers. Accessed June 2, 2021.
10. Vijayasarathi A, et al. Radiologists' online identities: what patients find when they search radiologists by name. AJR Am J Roentgenol 2016;207(5):952–8.
11. Calixto NE, et al. Factors impacting online ratings for otolaryngologists. Ann Otol Rhinol Laryngol 2018;127(8):521–6.

12. Carbonell G, et al. The use of recommendations on physician rating websites: the number of raters makes the difference when adjusting decisions. Health Commun 2019;34(13):1653–62.
13. Heimdal TR, et al. Factors affecting orthopedic sports medicine surgeons' online reputation. Orthopedics 2020;14:1–6.
14. Terlutter R, et al. Who uses physician-rating websites? Differences in sociodemographic variables, psychographic varibles, and health status of users and non-users of physician-rating websites. J Med Internet Res 2014;16(3):e97.
15. Callahan EJ, et al. The influence of patient age on primary care resident physician-patient interaction. J Am Geriatr Soc 2000;48(1):30–5.
16. Widmer RJ, et al. The impact of social media on negative online physician reviews: an observational study in a large, academic, multispecialty practice. J Gen Intern Med 2019;34(1):98–101.
17. Hawkins CM, et al. Social media and the patient experience. J Am Coll Radiol 2016;13:1615–21.
18. Dorfman RG, et al. Google ranking of plastic surgeons values social media presence over academic pedigree and experience. Aesthet Surg 2019;39(4):447–51.
19. Patient satisfaction- why it matters and how to improve it. Practice Builders; 2019. Available at: https://www.practicebuilders.com/blog/patient-satisfaction-why-it-matters-and-how-to-improve-it/. Accessed May 5, 2021.
20. What is patient experience? Agency for healthcare research and quality; 2021. Available at: https://www.ahrq.gov/cahps/about-cahps/patient-experience/index.html. Accessed May 5. 2021.
21. Institute of Medicine (US). Committee on quality of health care in America. Crossing the quality Chasm: a new health system for the 21st Century. Washington (DC): National Academies Press (US); 2001. Available at: https://www.ncbi.nlm.nih.gov/books/NBK222274/. Accessed May 5, 2021.
22. Fenton JJ, Jerant AF, Bertakis KD, et al. The cost of satisfaction. Arch Int Med 2012;172(5):405–11.
23. Borrelli M, Ting JY, Rabbani CC, et al. Patient satisfaction survey experience among American otolaryngologists. Am J Otolaryngol 2020;41(6):102656.
24. Picker.org. Influence, inspire, empower. Impact Report 2019-2020. Available at: https://www.picker.org/wp-content/uploads/2021/01/Picker_Impact-Report-2020_Web_spreads.pdf. Accessed May 2, 2021.
25. Patient satisfaction- why it matters and how to improve it. Practice builders; 2019. Available at: https://www.practicebuilders.com/blog/patient-satisfaction-why-it-matters-and-how-to-improve-it/. Accessed May 5, 2021.
26. Birkhäuer J, Gaab J, Kossowsky J, et al. Trust in the health care professional and health outcome: a meta- analysis. PLoS One 2017;12(2):e0170988.
27. PatientPop. 12 actionable ideas to improve patient experience. 2019. Available at: https://www.patientpop.com/blog/running-a-practice/patient-experience/ideas-to-improve-patient-experience/. Accessed May 2, 2021.
28. Albert Henry T. How to respond to bad online reviews. 2016. Available at: https://www.ama-assn.org/delivering-care/patient-support-advocacy/how-respond-bad-online-reviews. Accessed May 2, 2021.
29. Bacher R. How physicians can manage negative online reviews. 2018. Available at: https://www.enttoday.org/article/manage-negative-online-reviews/. Accessed May 2, 2021.

Coding for Optimal Payment (Correct Coding 2022 for Otolaryngology)

James Lin, MD[a],*, Richard W. Waguespack, MD[b]

KEYWORDS

- Current procedural terminology (CPT) • *ICD-10* • Coding • Billing • Business

KEY POINTS

- Business of Medicine, correct procedural coding, correct procedural reporting.
- Correct coding optimizes reimbursement and decreases chance of audit.
- CPT code usage is closely monitored and "squeezing" new procedures into pre-existing codes may lead to investigation and code family re-definition and revaluation
- Unlisted codes are not valued, but payers may reimburse for them if correctly requested in advance. As a corollary, the existence of a CPT codes does not guarantee payment.
- Several new code examples are provided in the manuscript.

CORRECT CODING IN OTOLARYNGOLOGY 2021

Proper billing of evaluation and management (E/M) encounters as well as procedural interactions with patients is of utmost importance across US health care. Incorrect reporting of E/M and current procedural terminology (CPT) codes can create differentials in reimbursement with drastic underpayment and overpayment compared with that associated with correct coding. To better understand the process of reimbursement by third-party payers, one may look to the origins of CPT. With the creation of Medicare in 1966, the US government opted to create a standardized method of reporting medical services to streamline the reimbursement process. This was tasked to the American Medical Association (AMA), and the CPT process was born. In 1992, Medicare sought to standardize reimbursement by creating the resource-based relative value scale (RBRVS), and the concept of the relative value unit (RVU) arose; this process is maintained by the AMA RBRVS Update Committee (RUC).

Conflicts of Interest: None.
[a] Department of Otolaryngology–Head and Neck Surgery, Kansas University Medical Center, 3901 Rainbow Boulevard, Mailstop 3010, Kansas City, KS 66160, USA; [b] Department of Otolaryngology–Head and Neck Surgery, The University of Alabama at Birmingham, Birmingham, AL 35294, USA
* Corresponding author.
E-mail address: Jlin2@kumc.edu

Otolaryngol Clin N Am 55 (2022) 137–144
https://doi.org/10.1016/j.otc.2021.07.010
oto.theclinics.com

Each CPT code is meant to represent a *distinct* service or procedure. Two types of CPT codes exist to report clinical services provided: category I and category III. The former are codes that we are most accustomed to reporting with higher literature support and widespread clinical use, whereas the latter do not require Food and Drug Administration (FDA) approval or high levels of evidence. Category III codes do not receive Medicare valuation but are used to track utilization of new procedures; despite this, they may be reimbursable by payers. As clinical practice evolves in Otolaryngology, new category I CPT codes are required, and existing ones may require revision or deletion. These processes occur with the input of Otolaryngologic societies via their CPT advisors to the AMA CPT Editorial Panel; the latter is the final determinant in dictating how a procedure is properly reported. Procedures and/or technology that differ from established ones will often require new CPT codes; before their establishment, the services will generally need to be submitted with unlisted codes. They are shepherded through the AMA CPT process primarily by specialty societies through a rigorous process of gathering and submitting information regarding incidence of condition or conditions treated in the United States, the prevalence of the procedure, and supporting literature regarding FDA clearance and efficacy of the novel procedure.

When a new CPT code is accepted or an existing one is revised, it is then referred to AMA RUC for valuation. Such valuation is based on surveys performed by specialty societies whose members perform the procedure and are presented to the RUC, a committee of physician delegates from varying specialties to determine the code value. Of note, RUC delegates who perform the service under investigation are not given the opportunity to deliberate on its valuation, and given Medicare's budget, adding value to codes often necessitates reduction to others. This valuation methodology highlights the need for survey respondents to provide input and be accurate and thoughtful in their responses. The nature of the process tends to decrease procedural values compared with E/M counterparts.

WHEN TO USE AN UNLISTED CODE

Very little is more confusing than use of unlisted codes. Correct coding does not allow use of an established code that only approximates the procedure performed. Existing codes are usually specific ("granular"), and this precision is carried into the valuation process in terms of RVUs. One must keep in mind that use of an unlisted code does not equate to nonreimbursement, and conversely, having a CPT code does not guarantee payment. When seeking reimbursement for an unlisted code, contact the payer in advance requesting preauthorization. Be specific regarding indications, provide literature support if needed, and fully delineate procedure work; provide comparison codes to justify the amount you are requesting. This will lead to payment delay, but if one does achieve coverage, future submissions should become more streamlined. On the other hand, once a procedure fulfills CPT criteria, an application to the panel may result in a reimbursable code. Private payers may still view new technology procedures with a CPT category I code to be "not medically necessary" and/or "experimental/investigational."

When using an unlisted code and the procedure performed encompasses one or more specific procedures in the same anatomic region that do have their own CPT code, use the unlisted code to describe the entirety of the procedure without a modifier, and do not report the component codes separately. Do use their valuation or valuations in your justification for reimbursement from the payer. CPT is looking to further refine the best practices for reporting unlisted with existing codes.

One may ask what the consequences might be for squeezing a procedure into a CPT code that approximates it? A personal pattern of using existing codes for another service may result in auditing and potentially being asked to return payments, or worse. Overall utilization of CPT codes is carefully monitored, and if meaningful changes occur (eg, increased frequency, different site of service), then specialty societies will be asked to explain the changes. This may result in a range of recommendations from increased education (by the specialty societies and AMA via *CPT Assistant*), resurvey of the code, or formal CPT code changes. It is important to remember that the ultimate authority for correct coding lies with the AMA CPT process, which is heavily dependent on medical specialty societies' input. The individual provider is ultimately responsible for charges that are submitted for services rendered.

OUTPATIENT EVALUATION AND MANAGEMENT

The codes remain the same (with exception of deleting 99201), but the criteria and values for outpatient E/M CPTs changed dramatically in 2021. At this writing, other types of E/M services (eg, observation, hospital) have not been modified in this fashion but are likely to undergo changes over the next several years. Not all payers may be aligned with these changes at present. The qualifying levels of history and examination have been removed from the E/M outpatient codes (only document relevant items), and only the degree of medical decision making (MDM), or total time, is considered. MDM addresses certain data, that is, diagnoses (number and severity), data reviewed, and risk of workup/treatment. A detailed description of the code changes may be found at https://www.ama-assn.org/system/files/2020-04/e-m-office-visit-changes.pdf[1]; also consult the introductory language in the current CPT book and *CPT Assistant* articles.

A thorough description of the changes is beyond the scope of this article, and there is no substitute for using a reference for these until your understanding and knowledge of the criteria are integrated into your workflow. How one documents the visit is of utmost importance in describing the acuity of the diagnoses treated, whether there is improvement, stability, or worsening of the problems. The number of records reviewed the day of service inclusive of notes from other providers, laboratory/pathology values, and imaging reports must also be documented. Either directly communicating with other providers to coordinate care or personally reviewing and independently interpreting test results and images also upgrades the level of complexity and must be captured in the note. Finally, the intervention and/or workup plans discussed with the patient must be documented, including specific risks for each. If the testing or imaging is already reported for reimbursement by the provider's practice, this does not count toward E/M data review complexity. An example is an audiogram performed and billed by a provider's practice; the provider cannot tally this as an "independent test."

Another question relates to the risks of workup and management, particularly the discussion of a "minor" versus a "major" procedure. A minor procedure is often considered to be one that has a global period of 10 days or less, whereas a major procedure has a global period that is longer, typically 90 days. The global period is the time after a procedure during which related, typical care is included in the overall procedure valuation. An average number of follow-up visits after a procedure, and their valuation for work and office equipment are accounted for in the total valuation of the CPT code. Most common global periods are 0, 10, and 90 days, although some payers may have different durations and reimbursement policies. It is important to be aware of the global periods associated with procedures to know when one can begin submitting charges again. For example, if a patient is within the global period of a procedure but has another, unrelated office visit (eg, sore throat evaluation within 90 days after a tympanoplasty), that encounter can be submitted for payment by appending the modifier 24 *Unrelated Evaluation and Management Service by the Same Physician or Other Qualified Health Care Professional During a Postoperative Period* to the E/M code.

Specific Coding Examples

Despite all the changes in outpatient E/M reporting, performing procedures in office and reporting them separately is still allowable with a −25 modifier appended to the E/M code. There have been growing attempts at discounting the E/M value up to 50% when the −25 modifier is appended by at least a handful of payers; however, the American Academy of Otolaryngology–Head and Neck Surgery/Foundation (AAO-HNS/F) has been successful in preventing these reductions from gaining a foothold thus far to remain consistent with the RBRVS framework.

Cerumen impaction has been defined by the AAO-HNS/F as "occurring when enough earwax accumulates to cause symptoms (pain, fullness, itching, odor, tinnitus, discharge, cough, or hearing loss), or to prevent needed assessment of the ear."[2] The typical code used to report cerumen disimpaction is 69210 to which a −50 (bilateral procedure) modifier may be appended. One should bear in mind that Centers for Medicare and Medicaid Services (CMS) and other payers may not recognize a −50 modifier with 69210 or even laterality with left (-LT) or right (-RT) modifiers, and use of these may impede reimbursement. Microscopy is no longer a prerequisite for reporting 69210; however, reporting binocular microscopy (92504) is typically not separately reimbursed for cerumen disimpaction. Documenting the nature of the impaction and instrumentation used for cerumen disimpaction is a prerequisite for reporting 69210. For lavage or irrigation of cerumen alone, use 69209. When performing cerumen disimpaction on the same day as an audiogram performed by the provider and/or provider's office, the proper code to report, particularly for Medicare patients, is G0268, which is inclusive of "one or both ears."

Flexible fiberoptic laryngoscopy (31575) is separately reportable with a −25 modifier appended to the E/M code if all elements of the latter are satisfied during the encounter. Like other in-office procedures, 31575 includes a brief history and review of results. If an encounter is cancer surveillance follow-up and nothing suggests exacerbation of disease or a new health issue, 31575 should be reported without a separate E/M code.

Eustachian tube balloon dilation (ETBD) is an example of a procedure receiving a CPT code but lacking coverage by some payers. After fulfilling criteria, 2 new category I CPT codes 69705 and 69706 for unilateral or bilateral eustachian tube dilation, respectively, were published. They have been valued for in-facility as well as office performance by CMS; however, not all payers consider the procedure to be medically necessary and are developing coverage policies on a payer-by-payer basis. Unlike sinus ostial dilation codes, these require the use of balloon dilation only and do not allow for dilation using nonballoon instrumentation. CPT codes 69705 and 69706 are inclusive of diagnostic nasal endoscopy (31231) and nasopharyngoscopy (92511), and these codes should not be reported separately. Also, the National Correct Coding Initiative (NCCI)[3–5] currently disallows reporting 69705 or 69706 with any surgical sinus procedure as well as several laryngoscopy, bronchoscopy, and esophagoscopy codes. The AAO-HNS at the time of publication is working to rectify this problem.

NCCI is a code edit ("bundling") process controlled ultimately by CMS to determine proper reimbursement for services deemed nonreportable together or to allow overrides in proper circumstances with modifiers (eg, 59 Distinct procedural service). Modifiers are discussed in more detail in later discussion. These are known as procedure-to-procedure (PTP) edits; an example would be reporting both unilateral and bilateral ETBD codes, 69705 and 69706, together. This is stated in CPT as a parenthetic instruction, and the edit disallowing simultaneous reporting cannot be bypassed. Other code pair edits may be appropriately overridden with modifier use when clinically appropriate. Lack of a PTP edit means the 2 procedures may be reported together for expected reimbursement. In addition, the NCCI also incorporates Medically Unlikely Edits (MUEs) that place limits on the number of times a procedure, device, or drug may be reimbursed for the same patient on the same day of service. For example, the MUE associated with tympanostomy tube placement is 2. CPT advisors for otolaryngology societies are typically asked to give feedback on proposed edits, but not always.

Another new CPT code is for placement of absorbable nasal implants for correction of nasal valve stenosis or collapse, 30468. Recently, technological advancements have led to the development of in-office or minimally invasive correction of nasal valve collapse, including implants, suture techniques, and scarification techniques. The performance of these new procedures led to miscoding with the traditional code for nasal valve stenosis repair, 30465. CPT code 30465 is defined and valued for a technique requiring incisions and direct placement with securing of grafts to correct nasal valve stenosis or collapse. Correct coding for minimally invasive nasal valve procedures was considered 30999, *Unlisted procedure, nose*. On further analysis, nasal valve collapse repair with absorbable nasal implants did meet the criteria for a category I code, and thus 30468 was adopted. However, because of a lack of literature support, other techniques involving scarification or nongraft suture techniques still require reporting with 30999. This is an example of the nuance relating to incorporating new technologies into the coding and reimbursement process. The reader is encouraged to update correct coding with future CPT material, such as the annual code book, *CPT Assistant* articles, specialty society publications, and timely attendance at coding education courses.

There have also been novel procedures developed for management of obstructive sleep apnea. In the diagnostic category is drug-induced sleep endoscopy (DISE), which is flexible transnasal endoscopy performed under anesthesia to simulate obstructive conditions to determine the site or sites of obstruction. At present, the recommended reporting of this procedure is with 31575, for flexible diagnostic laryngoscopy. Creating a code to incorporate the additional work and time spent performing DISE is currently under discussion. Similarly, the technology relating to hypoglossal nerve stimulation for the treatment of obstructive sleep apnea continues to evolve. Hypoglossal nerve stimulator placement is properly reported with CPT 64568, *Incision for implantation of cranial nerve (eg, vagus nerve) neurostimulator electrode array and pulse generator,* with add-on category III code 0466T, *insertion of respiratory chest wall sensor electrode or electrode array, including connection to the pulse generator.* When these procedures were initially reported, there was often denial of payment because the obstructive sleep apnea *International Classification of Diseases, Tenth Revision* (ICD-10) code, G47.33, was not a recognized indication for performing 64568. Also, CPT 0466T was only rarely reimbursed. Reimbursement for both 64568 and 0466T has become more widespread because of changes to payer policies. The higher levels of evidence in the literature and advocacy efforts of national, state, and local specialty and subspecialty otolaryngology societies with industry partners are the underpinnings for such positive coverage changes.

Tissue grafting and complex wound closure codes were updated in 2020. Free tissue grafting codes required updating because the now-deleted code 20926 was considered misvalued and was frequently being used inappropriately for reporting use of platelet-rich plasma. In addition, there were some issues regarding the work performed during liposuction-harvested fat grafting for reconstructive (noncosmetic) purposes. This led to formal discussions among stakeholder societies and development of 5 new codes for free tissue grafting, with 15769, *grafting of autologous soft tissue, other, harvested by direct excision*, which essentially replaced 20926. CPT codes 15771 to 15774 are used to report both liposuction-harvested fat and injection for reconstructive purposes. There is some confusion regarding the difference between 15769 and 15770, *graft derma-fat-fascia;* the delineating difference is that 15770 requires harvest of all 3 components: dermis, fat, *and* fascia, either en bloc or separately.

Complex wound closure codes have been updated because of ambiguity between intermediate (CPT codes 12031–12057) and complex (CPT codes 13100–13160) wound closure codes. The distinctions were delineated largely in the descriptive or introductory language of the code section in the Integumentary System. Whenever codes are changed, the reader should pay close attention not only to the code-specific descriptor language but also to parenthetic instructions beneath the codes and to general language regarding the code family.

The final specific topic of discussion in this article includes 2020 changes in computerized dynamic posturography coding that occurred primarily with increased utilization associated with CMS's decision to reimburse for 92548, *Computerized dynamic posturography* (old code descriptor before 2020). Several specialties (eg, audiology, neurology) had large increases in Medicare utilization of the code. This increased utilization was flagged and reviewed by the RUC, and it was determined that much of the reporting was inappropriate. Otolaryngology, neurology, and audiology societies were tasked with collaborating and clarifying the posturography code and submitting a code change application, which led to 2 new codes:

- 92548: *Computerized dynamic posturography sensory organization test, 6 conditions (ie, eyes open, eyes closed, visual sway, platform sway, eyes closed platform sway, platform and visual sway), including interpretation and report*
- 92549: *With motor control test and adaptation test*

Note that the posturography code expanded into a small code family with 92549 inclusive of the work of 92548 and extra testing. These code clarifications allow for reporting only if the provider used the appropriate posturography equipment and software, which are included in the codes' practice expense values.

In our discussions, we allude to the *CPT Assistant,* a monthly publication by the AMA that has an editorial board consisting of providers and coders whose role is to determine, with the aid of specialty CPT advisors, how difficult coding dilemmas are to be properly reported. It is tightly integrated with the CPT Editorial Panel and yet cannot answer questions that are ambiguous or not addressed in the code book. Such queries are often referred to the Panel for action. It provides timely guidance to queries and issues that may not be definitively answered in the annual CPT code book, as well as on new or modified codes.

Modifiers

Modifiers identify E/M and procedure codes for atypical circumstances. Proper use of modifiers 24 and 25 are discussed above. When performing a procedure on both sides on an anatomically described bilateral structure, append a −50 modifier, which typically reimburses at 150% of the allowable. To increase specificity regarding procedures on bilateral structures, report a left (-LT) or right (-RT) modifier when performed on 1 side alone. A difficult procedure owing to patient or anatomic factors may be appended with a −22 modifier *Increased procedural services*; however, when one reports this modifier, specific documentation is required to delineate the rationale for increased procedural work, time, and difficulty. When a patient is undergoing an urgent or emergent same-day major procedure, append a −57 modifier *Decision for surgery* to the E/M that includes the decision making resulting in the surgery. The −78 modifier *Unplanned Return to the Operating/Procedure Room by the Same Physician or Other Qualified Health Care Professional Following Initial Procedure for a Related Procedure During the Postoperative Period* is used when returning to the operating room for another procedure related to the original one, unplanned, during its global period (eg, obtaining hemostasis on a post–tonsillectomy bleed within a week). A −79 modifier *Unrelated Procedure or Service by the Same Physician or Other Qualified Health Care Professional During the Postoperative Period* is appended to a new procedure that is unrelated to the original procedure (eg, debridement of sinus surgery site after a combined septoplasty [global period 90 days] and endoscopic ethmoidectomy [global period of 0 days]). Appendix A of the CPT code book enumerates CPT modifiers.

Payer Policy

Throughout this discussion, the focus has been on correct coding, but there have also been references to payer policy, particularly used by private commercial insurers. This refers to how carriers reimburse for codes submitted. At a basic level, they will reimburse for services that are medically necessary and are considered covered services. Each company has its definition of medically necessary, but generally this refers to medical services that most reasonable practitioners feel are appropriate for the clinical situation being managed. Some covered services are simply not in the contract (eg, cosmetic procedures) or those which are considered experimental/investigational. This latter category includes services that the company feels do not have sufficient literature and/or widespread practitioner support to be considered clinically effective for the condition being managed and thus are not reimbursed. This does not mean it requires institutional review and is often applied to new technologies.

It is also important to link the proper *ICD-10* diagnostic code to its CPT counterpart, as a dissonance between the two may lead to payment denial. Payers generally link acceptable diagnoses to procedures and other services, so if the reported *ICD-10* is not on the list for a CPT code, then reimbursement may be denied. For example, chemodenervation of the larynx for patients with spasmodic dysphonia is generally a covered service, whereas using the same agent for a cosmetic condition likely is not; thus, linking the proper diagnosis with the corresponding CPT code is essential. Also, when using *ICD-10* codes, avoid those that are "unspecified," as payers have a tendency not to recognize them.

SUMMARY

Understanding rules of coding and discrepancies in valuation is demanding personally and when viewed strategically. At times, it may seem that negative valuation disparities exist among procedures, but attempting to address them with coding changes or via the RUC often has unintended and adverse consequences. If you find yourself asking for CPT code changes, especially involving new technology, be careful what you ask for. New codes that enter a family of existing codes risk revaluating the entire family, which may erode procedural values in comparison to E/M and similar services. Knowing how to properly code for clinical services optimizes safe reimbursement and minimizes risk of audit, monetary recoupment by payers, and even potential legal problems.

REFERENCES

1. Available at: https://www.ama-assn.org/system/files/2020-04/e-m-office-visit-changes.pdf. Accessed May 15, 2021.
2. Available at: https://www.entnet.org/content/aao-hnsf-clinical-practice-guideline-earwax-removal. Accessed May 15, 2021.
3. Available at: https://www.cms.gov/Medicare/Coding/NationalCorrectCodInitEd. Accessed May 15, 2021.
4. CPT 2021. Chicago: American Medical Association; 2021.
5. ICD-CM-2021. Chicago: American Medical Association; 2021.

E-Health and Telemedicine in Otolaryngology

Risks and Rewards

Lance A. Manning, MD[a,b,1], Christina M. Gillespie, MD[c,*]

KEYWORDS

- E-Health • Telehealth • Telemedicine • Business of medicine • Consultation
- Smart phones

KEY POINTS

- CMS has made significant changes to telemedicine rules in response to the current pandemic to allow doctors to safely care for patients.
- Smartphones, the Internet, and other advanced technology combined with sweeping changes to regulations has led to the wide adoption of telemedicine over the course of the last year.
- Telemedicine has the power to expand otolaryngologic services to underserved areas and populations.
- There are several challenges, including access to high-speed Internet, the need for special tools/technology, documentation, and patient privacy.
- Further improvements in technology could further expand the use of telemedicine in otolaryngology to include endoscopic examination, otologic examination, audiologic assessment, and speech therapy assessment from a remote setting.

INTRODUCTION

Telemedicine has been present in various progressive forms since the invention of the telegraph, the telephone, and radio transmission in the late nineteenth century. In the 1920s, an article published in *Science and Invention Magazine* by Hugo Gernsback heralded telehealth.[1] He described a device called a "teledactyl" that used radio communication that would allow doctors to see their patients through a viewscreen and touch them from miles away with spindly robot arms.[1] The rapidly changing communications landscape of the early twentieth century brought about the connectivity of

[a] Board of Governors, American Academy of Otolaryngology-Head and Neck Surgery; [b] Department of Otolaryngology, University of Arkansas for Medical Sciences; [c] Ocean Otolaryngology, 54 Bey Lea Road, Suite 3, Toms River, NJ 08753, USA
[1] Present address: 6823 Issacs Orchard, Springdale, AR 72762.
* Corresponding author. 2712 Lakewood Allenwood Road, Howell, NJ 07731
E-mail address: cmagillespie77@gmail.com
Twitter: @DrCGillespie (C.M.G.)

Otolaryngol Clin N Am 55 (2022) 145–151
https://doi.org/10.1016/j.otc.2021.07.011

the general population and the progression of the use of these technologies for remote medical access and practice. In the 1950s, radiologic images were transmitted via telephone, and in the 1960s, interactive two-way television was used to send physical examinations and provide distanced health services. However, it was not until the interconnectivity of the general population via the Internet in the late twentieth century that telehealth came into more widespread usage. Internet-based technological growth enabled the full potential of telehealth to start to be realized.[2] Although telemedicine was initially created as a way to treat patients in remote locations away from local health facilities or in areas with shortages of medical professionals, more recently it is increasingly used as a tool for convenient medical care and to limit patient contact, thus decreasing infectious disease risk.[2,3] As such, telemedicine implementation and use rapidly accelerated during the recent coronavirus disease 2019 (COVID-19) pandemic when lockdown restrictions limited patient care to virtual visits.[4] Rapid regulatory, legislative, and health insurance coverage changes ensued, which immediately expanded telemedicine services.[5–7] Between mid-March and mid-October 2020, more than 24.5 million out of 63 million Medicare beneficiaries and enrollees received a Medicare telemedicine service.[5]

DIFFERENCES BETWEEN TELEHEALTH, eHealth, AND TELEMEDICINE

With the interrelated fields of digital health, mobile health information technology, and telemedicine so frequently overlapping, the terms "telehealth" and "telemedicine" are often used interchangeably.[2] However, telemedicine is a more limited subset of telehealth. Telemedicine refers to delivering remote clinical services over a distance, such as medical education, remote patient monitoring, patient consultation via videoconferencing, wireless health applications, and transmission of imaging and medical reports.[8] Telehealth has a broader definition and can also include nonclinical activities, such as provider training, administrative meetings, continuing medical education, and public health functions. According to the World Health Organization, the term digital health is rooted in eHealth, which is defined as "the use of information and communications technology in support of health and health-related fields."[9] The World Health Organization further defines mobile health (mHealth) as a subset of eHealth and is defined as "the use of mobile wireless technologies for public health."[9] The term digital health was introduced as "…a term encompassing eHealth (which includes mHealth), as well as emerging areas, such as the use of advanced computing sciences in 'big data,' genomics and artificial intelligence."[9]

TELEHEALTH AND THE COVID-19 PANDEMIC

During the COVID-19 pandemic, there was an unprecedented adoption and use of telemedicine.[10] Many rapid regulatory, legislative, and health insurance coverage changes ensued with COVID-19. In February 2020, the Centers for Disease Control and Prevention issued guidance advising persons and health care providers in areas affected by the COVID-19 public health emergency to adopt social distancing practices, explicitly recommending that health care facilities and providers offer clinical services through virtual means, such as telehealth. On March 6, 2020, the Centers for Medicare & Medicaid Services announced telehealth policy changes and regulatory waivers in response to COVID-19. Telehealth provisions followed this as part of the US Coronavirus Aid, Relief, and Economic Security (CARES) Act, effective March 27, 2020.[11] These emergency policies included improved provider payments for telehealth, allowance for providers to serve out-of-state patients, authorization for multiple types of providers to offer telehealth services, reduced or waived cost-sharing for patients, and permission for federally qualified health centers or rural health clinics to provide telehealth services.[11] The waivers also allowed for virtual visits from the patient's home rather than in a health care setting.[11] During the COVID pandemic, several health policies and rates were temporarily altered at the federal and state level.[12] During that time, the Centers for Medicare & Medicaid Services increased telehealth reimbursement rates from $14 to $41, to $46 to $110 per visit.[12,13] Aetna, Anthem, Cigna, Humana, and United Healthcare also announced that they would pay physicians who conduct telehealth visits the same as their in-person rate in addition to paying claims for in-network and out-of-network physicians.[12]

As a result, there was an immediate increase in the number of telemedicine visits, with most encounters being from patients seeking care for conditions other than COVID-19.[11] There was a marked overall increase in the use of telehealth services and a concomitant sharp decline in the use of emergency departments.[11,14–16] These changes in telehealth were needed to increase access to patients. For various reasons, access to in-person health care was increasingly scarce. Patients with COVID19 could safely be cared for via telemedicine. Doctors' offices and clinics closed or severely reduced in-person capacity in response to safety concerns and stay-at-home orders. Additionally, patients avoided seeking in-person care during the pandemic. Overall, an estimated 41%–42% of US adults reported having delayed or avoided seeking care during the pandemic because of concerns about COVID-19, including 12% who reported having avoided seeking urgent or emergency care.[11,14–16] This rapid shift from in-person to virtual visits resulted in providers and patients gaining experience with telemedicine quickly. A study recently published by the American Academy of Otolaryngology-Head and Neck Surgery Telemedicine & Telehealth Working Group, found that of the survey respondents who answered questions about practice volume, 99% reported increased use of telemedicine during the pandemic.[4] Although telemedicine was generally well-accepted by patients and providers, this rapid expansion of telemedicine taught us all a great deal regarding its challenges, risks, limitations, and rewards.[4,11]

BENEFITS

Telemedicine demonstrated multiple rewards for individual and public health during the COVID-19 pandemic that continue to provide benefit. Remote screening and management of persons who needed clinical care for COVID-19 and other conditions increased access to care when many outpatient offices were closed or had limited operating hours.[11] The increased availability of telemedicine services reduced disease exposure for staff members and patients, preserved scarce supplies of personal protective equipment, and minimized patient surges on facilities.[11,17] In addition, many patients seeking telehealth in the early pandemic period were managed at home, which reduced large volumes of patients seeking care at health care facilities that were in the midst of a surge of COVID-19 cases.[11] Access to telehealth services was also valuable for patients who were reluctant to seek in-person care, had difficulty accessing in-person care, or had chronic conditions that placed them at high risk for severe COVID-19.[11]

Telemedicine has the power to break down geographic barriers to care access and allow patients with mobility issues to see providers from their homes. Telemedicine consultations can also allow for increased access to specialists in locations or facilities that are underserved. Additionally, increased telemedicine access can potentially reduce health care spending and such problems as medication nonadherence and unnecessary emergency room visits.[2]

The rewards of telemedicine extend beyond the COVID-19 pandemic. Telemedicine has the capacity to expand access to quality patient care, especially to remote rural regions and underserved populations.[2] Patients live in an increasingly technologically connected world. Telemedicine allows for a different kind of care experience.[2] With the increased access and flexibility for patients, patient convenience and engagement with telemedicine are rewards and driving forces.[2]

RISKS AND CHALLENGES OF TELEMEDICINE

Although there are multiple benefits in the judicious use of telemedicine, it is not without risks, challenges, and limitations. Several studies have shown that the socio-economic status of a country, and an individual, can limit telemedicine access and feasibility.[18,19] It has been clear that much of the limited access to telemedicine is related to limited access to the Internet or technology devices, such as computers, smartphones, or tablets.[11,20] Additionally, unfamiliarity with technology or disabilities that limit or prohibit the use of these technologies are potential barriers for some patients.[11,20] In addition, virtual visits might not be best for some persons based on level of medical acuity or necessity to conduct an in-person physical examination or diagnostic testing.[11]

Telemedicine platforms require training, software and possibly equipment purchases.[2] Additionally, more extensive inpatient telemedicine platforms used between doctors requesting consultations and consulting specialists usually require more training and the purchase of a telemedicine cart and various mobile health devices.[2]

The scalability of telemedicine opens the door for on-demand care from consumer-facing companies, where a patient can log in and request a visit with a random provider. However, that provider likely does not know the patient nor has the ability to have the patient follow-up with them in person should the visit necessitate a physical examination.

In otolaryngology, a thorough examination of regions that require specific tools, such as the ears, nose, sinuses, and throat, is difficult to conduct remotely. Additionally, palpation by the clinician to examine structures is not available via telemedicine encounters, thus delaying diagnosis of a known or occult mass. Other medical specialties that do not require as much patient touch or direct examination of luminal structures may be more amenable to telemedicine, such as teleradiology, telepathology, telepsychiatry, and teledermatology. However, new technology could greatly expand the use of telemedicine in otolaryngology. Otolaryngology can be adapted to telemedicine because of the use of endoscopic images and videos. Tools can be developed to be used in the remote office or even at home to allow improved visualization. Also, smartphones are revolutionizing telemedicine. Smartphones may be used one day for a variety of applications, such as screening for hearing loss and voice analysis. Further validation and study are needed before widespread adoption of endoscopic and smartphone applications in telemedicine.

With the use of new technologies for telemedicine, clinicians face challenges following the usual protocols, quality assurance, and institutional norms.[21] Continued appropriate documentation, follow-up, adverse event reporting, and patient privacy protocols must be observed.

TYPES OF TELEMEDICINE CONSULTATIONS

There are three primary types of telemedicine: (1) remote monitoring, (2) store-and-forward, and (3) real-time interactive visits.[22] Remote monitoring also includes self-testing and self-monitoring and uses a range of technologies to monitor patients remotely. This type of telemedicine is used extensively to manage some chronic diseases, such as asthma, diabetes mellitus, and cardiovascular disease.

Store-and-forward or "asynchronous" telemedicine uses stored information, such as images, laboratory results, recorded videos, or history reports, which is sent to a physician at a different location who need not be communicating with the patient at the same time. This type of telemedicine is common in the fields of dermatology, pathology, and radiology.[22]

Real-time or "synchronous" telemedicine services are live interactions between a health care provider and a patient or another provider and offer a virtual alternative to an in-person visit. This is accomplished via audio-only, video, or both using a variety of communication devices. There are constantly changing regulations and insurance payer policies with regards to how these services are reimbursed. Again, providers should check with their respective payers to confirm authorizations of reimbursable telemedicine services and restrictions on the site requirements of the patient and the provider.

LICENSURE AND MALPRACTICE CONSIDERATIONS

If one is licensed in the state where the patient is located, there are generally no additional telemedicine licensure requirements. If one is not licensed in the state where the patient is located, the circumstance varies according to the state where the physician and the patient are located.[23] During the COVID-19 pandemic, Centers for Medicare & Medicaid Services issued waivers for Medicare patients, temporarily waiving requirements that out-of-state providers be licensed in the state where they are providing services when they are licensed in another state. Physicians are still bound by their state licensing requirements.[24]

Many states have temporarily relaxed licensure requirements related to physicians licensed in another state and retired or clinically inactive physicians.[23] This includes waiving licensure requirements or offering a temporary expedited license for out-of-state physicians. Many but not all of these measures apply to physicians providing telemedicine across state lines. Additionally, since the COVID-19 pandemic, there has been significant growth in the number of states participating in the Interstate Medical Licensure Compact.[25] This is an agreement among participating US states to work together to significantly streamline the licensing process for physicians who want to practice in multiple states. Please contact your state board of medicine or department of health for up-to-the-minute information. Regarding medical malpractice insurance considerations, check with your malpractice insurance carrier to ensure your policy covers providing care via telemedicine. Malpractice insurance carriers may not cover multiple states and often must be notified when out-of-state consultation is contemplated.

There is also variability between states with respect to requiring health care providers to obtain informed consent to use telemedicine.[2] Whether or not a state requires this, it is always good practice for providers. One should consider explaining the telemedicine protocols and policies for virtual visits, prescribing, and care coordination and any limits on patient confidentiality.[2]

SUMMARY

In the wake of the catastrophic impact of COVID-19, innovative solutions and implementation in telemedicine have created a transformation in health care.[18] The response to the pandemic provided a unique opportunity to see the role that telemedicine can play in health care. With the resultant expanded access, improved reimbursement policies, and acceptance by patients and health care providers, telemedicine will likely serve as an important modality for delivering care even after the pandemic.[11] There is compelling evidence to suggest that telehealth may have a significant effect on advancing health care in the future.[18] In otolaryngology, this can certainly serve as an adjunct to in-person care to increase patient convenience, access, and engagement. Because the head and neck region's unique anatomy often requires palpation and specific tools to examine and surgically treat luminal structures in the ears, nose, and throat, today's available technology limits how much of the scope of otolaryngology can presently be performed remotely.

DISCLOSURE

The authors have nothing to disclose.

REFERENCES

1. Novak M. Telemedicine predicted in 1925. In Smithsonian Magazine. Available at: https://www.smithsonianmag.com/history/. Accessed May 9, 2021.
2. What is telemedicine? In: eVisit Resources. 2021. Available at: https://evisit.com/resources/what-is-telemedicine/. Accessed May 9, 2021.
3. Understanding telehealth. Available at: https://telehealth.hhs.gov/patients/understanding-telehealth/. Accessed May 9, 2021.
4. Levi JR, Yu VX, Cheung AY, et al. Tele-otolaryngology: through the pandemic, and beyond-interim findings of the study of telehealth in otolaryngology. In Bulletin-The official member magazine of the American Academy of Otolaryngology-Head and Neck Surgery. May 2021; Vol. 40, No. 4.
5. Trump Administration Finalizes. Permanent expansion of Medicare telehealth services and improved payment for time doctors spend with patients. Newsroom, CMS.gov. December. 2020. Available at: https://www.cms.gov/newsroom/press-releases/trump-administration-finalizes-permanent-expansion-medicare-telehealth-services-and-improved-payment. Accessed May 9, 2021.
6. CY 2021 Medicare physician fee schedule final rule. 2021. Available at: https://www.cms.gov/medicaremedicare-fee-service-paymentphysicianfeeschedpfs-federal-regulation-notices/cms-1734-f. Accessed May 10, 2021.
7. Telehealth: delivering care safely during COVID-19. U.S. Department of Health & Human Services. 2020. Available at: https://www.hhs.gov/coronavirus/telehealth/index.html. Accessed May 9, 2021.
8. Gajarawala S, Pelkowski J. Telehealth benefits and barriers. J Nurse Pract 2020; 17(2):218–21.
9. World Health Organization. Guideline recommendations on digital interventions for health system strengthening. Geneva (Switzerland): World Health Organization; 2019.
10. Holtz BE. Patients perceptions of telemedicine visits before and after the coronavirus disease 2019 pandemic. Telemed E-Health 2021;27:1.
11. Trends in the use of telehealth during the emergence of the COVID-19 pandemic—United States, January–March 2020. Centers for Disease Control and Prevention. MMWR Morb Mortal Wkly Rep 2020;69:1595–9.
12. Moore MA, Munroe DD. Opinion: COVID-19 brings about rapid changes in the telehealth landscape. Telemed E-Health 2021;27:4.
13. Twachtman G. CMS hike telephone payments during the pandemic. Medscape 2020. Available at: https://www.cms.gov/newsroom/press-releases/trump-

administration-issues-second-round-sweeping-changes-support-us-healthcare-system-during-covid. Accessed May 9, 2021.

14. Mehrotra A, Chernew M, Linetsky D, et al. The impact of the COVID-19 pandemic on outpatient visits: a rebound emerges. New York: Commonwealth Fund; 2020. Available at: https://www.commonwealthfund.org/publications/2020/apr/impact-covid-19-outpatient-visits.

15. Hartnett KP, Kite-Powell A, DeVies J, et al. National Syndromic Surveillance Program Community of Practice. Impact of the COVID-19 pandemic on emergency department visits—United States, January 1, 2019–May 30, 2020. MMWR Morb Mortal Wkly Rep 2020;69:699–704.

16. Czeisler MÉ, Marynak K, Clarke KEN, et al. Delay or avoidance of medical care because of COVID-19–related concerns—United States, June 2020. MMWR Morb Mortal Wkly Rep 2020;69:1250–7.

17. Larry A. Green Center. Quick COVID-19 primary care survey, series 3, fielded March 27–30, 2020. Richmond (VA): Larry A. Green Center; 2020.

18. Doraiswamy S, Abraham A, Mamtani R, et al. Use of telehealth during the COVID-19 pandemic: scoping review. J Med Internet Res 2020;22(12):e24087.

19. Barry-Menkhaus SA, Wagner DV, Stoeckel M, et al. Socioeconomic factors: access to and use of diabetes technologies. In: Klonoff DC, Kerr D, Mulvaney SA, editors. Diabetes digital health. Netherlands: Elsevier; 2020. p. 145–55.

20. Reed ME, Huang J, Graetz I, et al. Patient characteristics associated with choosing a telemedicine visit vs. office visit with the same primary care clinicians. JAMA Netw Open 2020;3:e205873.

21. Bashshur R, Doarn CR, Frenk JM, et al. Telemedicine and the COVID-19 pandemic, lessons for the future. Telemed E-Health 2020;26:5.

22. Smith Y. Types of telemedicine. In: News Medical. 2021. Available at: https://www.news-medical.net/health/Types-of-Telemedicine.aspx. Accessed May 10, 2021.

23. Federation of State Medical Boards. U.S. states and territories modifying requirements for telehealth in response to COVID-19. 2021. Available at: https://www.fsmb.org/siteassets/advocacy/pdf/states-waiving-licensure-requirements-for-telehealth-in-response-to-covid-19.pdf. Accessed May 10, 2021.

24. Centers for Medicare and Medicaid Services. Fact sheets & frequently asked questions (FAQs). 2021. Available at: https://www.cms.gov/CCIIO/Resources/Fact-Sheets-and-FAQs. Accessed May 10, 2021.

25. Robeznieks A. Cross-state licensing process now lives in 30 states. The American Medical Association. Apr 2021. Available at: https://www.ama-assn.org/practice-management/digital/cross-state-licensing-process-now-live-30-states. Accessed May 10, 2021.

Malpractice Woes
Here Is What You Should Do if You Get Sued

Stephen P. Cragle, MD[a], Garin L. Strobl, JD[b],*

KEYWORDS

- Medical malpractice • Lawsuit • Claim • CANDOR • Apology • Anxiety

KEY POINTS

- Being involved in a medical malpractice claim or lawsuit can leave a lasting mark on a provider and can be accompanied by feelings of shame, isolation, anger, and anxiety.
- There are several things a provider can do to make the process of a medical malpractice matter easier: get support, be engaged, and give yourself grace.
- Communication with patients can be a key aspect in preventing a medical malpractice situation, including apologizing to the patient after an adverse event.

INTRODUCTION

Medical malpractice actions are far from rare: 34% of physicians practicing in 2016 reported being sued. Incidences of reported malpractice suits ranged from 8% of physicians under age 40 to 49% of physicians aged 50 and older. Rates were highest among emergency physicians, general surgeons, obstetricians/gynecologists, and surgical subspecialists. Of surgical subspecialists over the age of 55, 67% report having been sued.[1]

Most physicians named in malpractice suits prevail: 68% of suits are dropped, 23% result in settlements, 6% result in verdicts for the defendant (physician), and 1% for the plaintiff.[2] A physician facing a malpractice lawsuit can expect to ultimately prevail in 3 out of 4 cases, whether by dismissal or a favorable verdict, but at what cost? Financial pressures, schedule disruption, mood disorders, burnout, and family stress often accompany a lawsuit. Feelings of shame and fear of being pejoratively labeled assail most physicians who find themselves in this stressful situation. One of the authors has personally had the misfortune of encountering this unpleasant experience twice in a 29-year career: once in residency and again in practice just a few years ago.

[a] St. Cloud Ear, Nose & Throat Clinic, P.A., 1528 Northway Drive, St. Cloud, MN 56303, USA;
[b] Constellation Mutual, 7701 France Avenue, Suite 500, Minneapolis, MN 55435, USA
* Corresponding author.
E-mail address: garin.strobl@constellationmutual.com
Twitter: @docsadvice (S.P.C.)

Otolaryngol Clin N Am 55 (2022) 153–160
https://doi.org/10.1016/j.otc.2021.07.012
0030-6665/22/© 2021 Elsevier Inc. All rights reserved.

MALPRACTICE LAWSUIT: A SURGEON'S PERSPECTIVE

In 1991, as a senior resident in otolaryngology/head and neck surgery at the University of Wisconsin Hospitals and Clinics, I was named in a lawsuit along with my attending and 2 other residents. I rounded on the patient and discussed care with my colleagues, but did not take an active part in their treatment. The case was interesting but unremarkable, and the patient had a good outcome. At the time, I was bewildered by the lawsuit, because a dentist and a primary care physician failed to diagnose correctly, and the patient presented to us with a complicated history that we untangled, diagnosed, and treated with a good resolution of their symptoms. Ultimately, the case was dismissed because the plaintiff could not find an expert to challenge the appropriateness of the care.

Over the 2 or 3 years from first receiving notice of legal action to the dismissal, I experienced several bouts of anxiety, fear (for my future in practice), and anger toward the plaintiff, who I viewed as unfair and ungrateful. Although the lawsuit was dismissed, I was subjected to scrutiny for several years in the form of reporting requirements for every medical staff and other professional application thereafter to recount the details of that event. I truly feared that I would be declined for medical staff and other appointments based on the shameful status of having been named in a legal action. I remember to this day with eerie clarity the patient's name, appearance, family, and even the appearance of the computed tomography slice that identified the pathology. I had a great deal of mental anguish despite my conviction that the care our team delivered was both timely and standard of care.

I suffered silently; only my spouse and my office administrator knew of the event. I neither sought nor was offered any counseling, and I made no effort to discuss my private struggles with my clinic partners, who I assumed would judge me either for seeking help or for getting sued in the first place. I probably became somewhat more defensive and conservative in my otolaryngology practice, although I quickly put the trauma behind me and began to really enjoy my career.

Twenty-five years later, in 2016 I received a notice from a local plaintiff's attorney that I was named in a lawsuit filed by a patient that I operated on in 2013. Again, I remember the patient, their presentation, and the procedure with crystal clarity. The patient sought care for a painful neck swelling and seemed depressed and anxious about their condition. I recommended a surgical procedure, but the patient implored me to do a more minimally invasive approach and, against my better judgment, I agreed. The procedure was unsuccessful and resulted in additional pain and swelling. After again offering the original procedure, the patient sought treatment elsewhere and underwent the offered procedure there successfully. I did not hear from them afterward until their attorney mailed the notice.

I had communicated with the patient on several occasions during their treatment interval with me. Discussion of risks, benefits, and alternatives for the procedure was carried out as standard of care. I empathized with the patient's condition without implying culpability. In retrospect, I believe that my only error was in acquiescing to their wish for a less invasive approach, which I was uncertain would treat their condition.

After I received the lawsuit notification, I contacted my malpractice insurance company who assigned Garin Strobl, JD, my coauthor for this article. I confessed to her that I was fearful, anxious, and angry about the accusations brought by the plaintiff, and went on to describe the case from my point of view. She listened carefully and began to outline her plan for the case. She carefully detailed the legal process, the likely timeline, what was expected of me, and what I could expect from the legal team. I felt both validated and reassured. She then explained that a counselor would call me to help with my emotional turmoil. After several conversations with the counselor, I felt like I had a better understanding of my emotions and better equilibrium for continuing my practice and my day-to-day life. Our defense team decided the case merited refusal of any settlement and determination to try the case if necessary. After many months, the plaintiff's attorney chose to allow the case to be dismissed, again for lack of any expert to challenge the appropriateness of care.

As I compare 2 very similar events that form a pair of bookends to my career so far, I am struck by the different pathway I was offered in each case. In the earlier event, I was pretty much left to figure out my own way to process the hurt, fear, and anxiety; in the latter, I was given resources that materially improved my mental health and decreased the stress associated with an already stressful event. In this article, we hope to dispel confusion about the process of defending against a lawsuit or civil action, and offer resources to reduce anxiety, cynicism, and feelings of burnout that often accompany the process.

GETTING SUPPORT DURING A MEDICAL MALPRACTICE EVENT: AN ATTORNEY'S PERSPECTIVE

As you can see from these comments, being involved in a medical malpractice claim or lawsuit can stay with a provider forever. Attorneys frequently speak with doctors who, decades later, still remember every detail about the care of a patient who brought a medical malpractice action. Providers also often tell me that the memory of an old claim or lawsuit will reemerge years later when seeing a patient for an issue that was similar to the one involved in the prior claim or lawsuit. Some providers carry the burden of dealing with a medical malpractice case without even telling their families; for a small minority, it has driven them to leave the practice.

Stress from a medical malpractice event is so common that there's actually a diagnosis for it: medical malpractice stress syndrome.[3] The first step for providers is to accept that medical malpractice claims and lawsuits are stressful, and then to seek out support. For some practitioners, that might just mean talking with a spouse or colleague; for others, it might involve mental health therapy or support from a religious leader. Whatever form it takes, getting support helps providers to get back to doing the most important things: providing good care to their patients and taking care of themselves.

The good news is that both employers and medical malpractice carriers are recognizing the stress that accompanies these experiences and are providing resources to help. Some health care groups have a designated team of providers who are on hand to support the provider. Support is often less formal in smaller organizations, where the administrator might serve as a source of support. There might also be another provider in the group who has encountered the same experience and is able to provide guidance and a listening ear. Your medical malpractice carrier might also have support resources in place. Whatever approach you prefer, I have never had a doctor tell me that he or she regretted having support during this stressful and difficult time. In a role where you are always helping others, sometimes asking for help for yourself can make all the difference.

LITIGATION TIMELINE: WHAT TO EXPECT

Many providers are surprised to learn that a medical malpractice lawsuit will likely last several years from the time you receive the summons and complaint to when the jury reaches its verdict.[4] What can make the process even more frustrating is that there may be several months where it seems like there's been no activity with the case. Each state has a different process for medical malpractice cases, but they typically fall into the following phases: lawsuit initiation, discovery, and the trial.

Lawsuit Initiation

The first step of a lawsuit is receiving the initial legal paperwork from the plaintiff, called the complaint. This document typically contains a lot of boilerplate language and, depending on the attorney, may not provide much substantive information about the allegations. Some states allow plaintiffs to proceed directly to court, whereas others require that the plaintiff start his or her case with a medical review panel. Contact your medical malpractice carrier as soon as you receive a complaint, because you will only have a certain time to respond, and you might face consequences for missing a response deadline.

Discovery

This phase of the lawsuit is when information is shared between the parties. Each side has the ability to exchange written questions. This phase also includes depositions of the parties and, depending on the state, the expert witnesses. By this point in the lawsuit, your attorney will likely have completed the expert reviews on your behalf, and you will have an idea of whether your case is defensible either because you have support for the standard of care, causation, or hopefully, both. Your attorney and insurer will work with you to discuss any concerns that may have arisen during the expert reviews and whether they believe your case is defensible. If they believe your case is not defensible, they will suggest trying to resolve the case through a settlement.

Trial

The trial is typically the most stressful time of the litigation process. You should plan to be present for the entire duration of the trial. Depending on the complexity of the case, the trial could last for a few days or several weeks. It is important to make sure you are getting the support you need during this difficult phase. The hardest part of the trial is the beginning, when the plaintiff gets to present their case. You will have to sit in front of a jury while the plaintiff's medical experts testify against you, and the plaintiff and their family testify about what you allegedly did, and the effects it has had on their lives. Once the plaintiff concludes their presentation, your attorney will present your side of the story. You likely will testify, and the jury will also hear from the medical experts who are on your side. Once the defense wraps up, the case will go to the jury for deliberation. Some deliberations last only a matter of hours, whereas others last for days. The odds are in your favor; in recent years, plaintiffs have won only 23% of medical malpractice cases.[5]

WHAT TO DO IF YOU GET SUED

Providers can take several steps to help make a medical malpractice lawsuit easier: be engaged, trust the process, and give yourself grace.

Be Engaged

The more engaged a provider is in his or her medical malpractice event, the better. Avoiding the process—by not reading emails from defense counsel or inadequately preparing for your deposition—will only make your position worse and more stressful. Furthermore, both your defense counsel and medical malpractice carrier are looking for your thoughts throughout the claim or the suit because you are their expert and are in the best position to provide an opinion on some of the medical components, and what the other side's experts might be saying. And do not be afraid to ask questions. Your defense attorney and insurer are there to help make the process as transparent as possible. They would rather have you ask questions as they arise than withhold those questions until they fester and add to your stress. The more you stay involved in the process, the fewer surprises you will encounter along the way.

Trust the Process

Medical treatments are your expertise; malpractice claims and litigation are where your attorney and carrier are experts. Just like your defense attorney would never tell you how to perform a surgery or how to diagnose a patient, you should have faith that your defense attorney and malpractice carrier know what they are doing when it comes to a malpractice issue. Most medical malpractice carriers use an approved panel of attorneys who have been chosen because they focus their practice on medical malpractice cases and have a proven track record of success. Litigating a medical malpractice case can be a complex process and your medical malpractice team will be constantly evaluating your case to get you the best resolution possible. This might mean settling the case if they cannot find support for the care, or, in many cases, taking the case to trial because you provided good care. Your defense attorney and medical malpractice carrier also will be looking for opportunities to have the case against you dismissed if they can, but unfortunately, those opportunities can be rare. Whatever the route a malpractice issue might take, know that your defense attorney and insurance carrier will keep you advised on the best course of action.

Give Yourself Grace

Providers often blame themselves when they are the subject of a medical malpractice situation. They replay the situation constantly in their heads and think about everything they should have done to prevent the outcome. One of the reasons a medical malpractice situation can be difficult on a provider is that you usually know the end of the story: there may have been a missed diagnosis or an atypical anatomy that led to an adverse outcome in a surgery. It is always easy to work backward and think, "I should have known about X, that would have prevented this outcome." But as the saying goes, hindsight is 20/20, and it is important to remember that you may not have had all the information available to you at the time. Or, even if you did, you still acted reasonably in the circumstance. The standard of care that matters in malpractice lawsuits is the level of care that a reasonably competent medical provider, in similar circumstances (ie, same practice area and a similar medical community), would have provided under the circumstances. In a basic sense, the standard of care is providing reasonable care based on the information you had at the time. If you are faced with a medical malpractice claim or lawsuit, give yourself grace, and remember that you likely acted within the standard of care even though the care may not seem perfect in retrospect when you are faced with detailed allegations from the other side.

APOLOGY AND COMMUNICATION AFTER AN ADVERSE EVENT

From time to time, we will get questions about how to avoid a medical malpractice situation. There is obviously no way to guarantee you will never be faced with this situation, and some specialties are more at risk than others,[6] but one of the biggest things a provider can do to maintain a good relationship with his or her patient, and possibly prevent a malpractice event, is be a good communicator.[7] Years ago, health care providers were taught never to apologize to patients after an adverse event based on the concern that the apology could be used as an admission of liability. As a result, patients and their families understandably believed that a provider and his or her employer were not communicating because they were trying to cover up wrongdoing. The end result was that everyone suffered: the patient and family struggled with the aftermath of an adverse event, and the provider felt horrible that his or her patient experienced an adverse event and the provider could not discuss it with them and show empathy.

Luckily, conventional wisdom has changed for the better, and providers now are having these conversations with patients. A majority of states already have some sort of legislation that prohibits certain forms of apologies from being used against the provider in court,[8] and some states have even created Communication and Optimal Resolution (CANDOR) laws, which offer certain protections to providers who engage in these discussions with patients and their families. Colorado is one of the few states that has enacted a CANDOR law that allows a provider to share how the situation happened, and what changes will be made to prevent future instances. These discussions—and any offers of compensation—are privileged and confidential.[9] Patients who decide to engage in the CANDOR process in Colorado still have the right to pursue a lawsuit. However a study out of Michigan, which also has a CANDOR law, showed that medical claims dropped by more than one-half for one of the state's health care systems.[10] Contact your medical malpractice carrier if a situation arises where an apology might be warranted, because they may be able to assist you in facilitating the discussion.

MALPRACTICE: IMPLICATIONS FOR OTOLARYNGOLOGISTS

The most frequent otolaryngology cases implicated in malpractice actions include orbital complications of endoscopic sinus surgery, facial nerve injuries in parotid surgery, recurrent laryngeal nerve injuries in thyroid surgery, and post-tonsillectomy hemorrhage complications. Questions of medical necessity, compliance with published guidelines, and failure to achieve adequate informed consent form the bulk of the reasons for initiating a malpractice action. (Dr Kmucha is a practicing Otolaryngologist with a law degree who has written extensively on malpractice and other legal topics of interest to Otolaryngologists).

When cases with a jury verdict are examined, rhinologic cases—especially endoscopic sinus surgery—generally comprise the largest segment of these actions against otolaryngologists, followed by head and neck surgery and facial plastic surgery. Improper surgical performance, failure to diagnose, refer, or treat, and informed consent issues comprise the main issues in these cases. Of jury verdicts, 82% to 89% ruled in favor of the otolaryngologist.[11]

Clinical practice guidelines perform a useful function to guide clinical decision-making, and otolaryngologists should be familiar with applicable clinical practice guidelines when tailoring a treatment plan for each patient. When a particular patient's care requires significant deviation from the appropriate guideline, documenting the reasons for the deviation as well as the appropriate discussion with the patient may decrease legal risk in the case of an unexpected complication.[12]

Over the past few decades, otolaryngology paid claims per capita has dropped, whereas the average claim paid has increased: from 1992 to 2014, there were 24.4 paid claims per year per 1000 physician-years. From 1992 to 1996 the rate was 33.0 and for 2009 to 2014 it was 16.4, decreasing by 50.3% over a 20-year period.[13] This pattern mirrored most other surgical subspecialties, as well as physicians in general. Average payments per claim and the percentage of catastrophic claims paid increased significantly in the same period. Possible reasons for the decrease in paid claims include tort reform efforts; improvement in patient safety with checklists, time-outs, and handoffs; corporate "shielding" of individual physicians by hospital systems to avoid reporting to the National Practitioner Data Base; and alternative resolution programs that do not require a written claim from a patient. Possible reasons for the increase in payment per claim include reticence by plaintiffs' attorneys to bring smaller claims because of the potential for loss and increased administrative burden; pretrial screening panels for the same reason; or settling smaller claims outside the written claims process, leaving only larger claims in the database.[14]

SUMMARY

Even with optimal care, medical malpractice risks are part of the practice of otolaryngology. There are many ways to safeguard yourself and your practice from these unpleasant events, but even when all precautions have been taken and every effort has been made to choose the best treatment option together with your patient, you might still find yourself facing a malpractice suit. Take a deep breath, remember that you are not alone, and do not despair. Seek help from your employer, medical malpractice insurer, and family, and take the steps outlined in this article to help make the situation better. You might just find light at the end of the tunnel, and renewed joy in your practice if you do.

DISCLOSURE

The authors have nothing to disclose.

REFERENCES

1. Guardado JR. Policy research perspectives: medical liability claim frequency among U.S. physicians. American Medical Association; 2017. Available at: https://www.ama-assn.org/media/21976/download.
2. Guardado JR. Policy research perspectives: medical professional liability insurance indemnity payments, expenses and claim disposition, 2006-2015. American Medical Association; 2018. Available at: https://www.ama-assn.org/media/21966/download.
3. Scibilia J. Medical malpractice stress syndrome can affect physical, mental health. Medical malpractice stress syndrome. AAP News; 2020. Available at: https://www.aappublications.org/news/2020/08/01/wellness080120.
4. Jena AB, Chandra A, Lakdawalla D, et al. Outcomes of Medical Malpractice Litigation Against US Physicians. Arch Intern Med 2012;172(11):892–4.
5. Lee C, LaFountain R. Medical malpractice litigation in state courts. Natl Cent St Cts 2011;18:1–7.
6. American Osteopathic Society. Available at: https://thedo.osteopathic.org/2019/12/physicians-in-these-10-specialties-are-most-likely-to-get-sued-by-a-patient/. Accessed April 17, 2021.
7. Medical schools have recognized the importance of good communication, and now most medical schools include communication skills in their programs. In: Mauksch LB, Arnold RW, Losh DP, et al. Teaching inpatient communication skills to medical students: an innovative strategy. Acad Med 2005; 18:118-124.
8. Gallegos A. Candor laws growing, but are they effective? Clin Neurol 2016; 17(3):1–18.

9. Martin J. An overview of the Colorado Candor Act. In: Colorado medical Society. 2019. Available at: https://www.cms.org/articles/an-overview-of-the-colorado-candor-act. Accessed April 17, 2021.

10. The Michigan model: medical malpractice and patient safety at Michigan Medicine. In: Michigan Medicine: University of Michigan. Available at: uofmhealth.org/michigan-modelmedical-malpractice-and-patient-safety-umhs. Accessed April 18, 2021.

11. Svider PF, Husain Q, Kovalerchik O, et al. Determining legal responsibility in otolaryngology: a review of 44 trials since 2008. Am J Otolaryngol 2013;34(6): 699–705.

12. Ruhl DS, Siegal G. Medical malpractice implications of clinical practice guidelines. Otolaryngol Head Neck Surg 2017;157(2):175–7.

13. Schaffer AC, Jena AB, Seabury SA, et al. Rates and characteristics of paid malpractice claims among US physicians by specialty, 1992-2014. JAMA Intern Med 2017;177(5):710–8.

14. Breen CT, Mehra S. An analysis of otolaryngology medical malpractice payments from the national practitioner data bank. Otolaryngol Head Neck Surg 2021; 164(3):589–94.

Organizing a Successful Practice and Considering Tax and Estate Planning

Lawton C. Leung, AB, JD, LLM[a], K.J. Lee, MD[b,c,d,e,*], Alexander Jin[f]

KEYWORDS

- Building successful practice • Tax planning • Estate planning

KEY POINTS

- Building successful practice.
- Tax and estate planning.
- Skills to treat, heart to care.

ORGANIZING A SUCCESSFUL PRACTICE

To care for your family and to do "good" for your alma mater, religious organization, and the other charities you love, you need to do "well," which is to build a successful practice. To achieve a successful practice, following the principles of the dozen A's is helpful: Ability, Availability, Amicability, Approachable, Attuned, Aware, Attentive to patients, Attentive to others, Attentive to details, Apology (ability to apologize and accept apology gracefully), Assimilate, Affordable. Another way to put it is "skills to treat, heart to care at a sensible price."

Ability is for one to keep up with the latest in medicine and technology in the specialty and know your own limitations. Strive to get the best outcome and experience for your patients and encourage them to seek a second opinion. Treat every patient as if you or your loved one is the patient. In 2016, I founded a nonprofit foundation called *The Patient Is U*, Inc ("TPIU") to "[d]o unto others what you want others to do unto you."

Pay attention to 2 components: the organization (the office) and the doctor. From the organization standpoint, install the right protocols and technology as well as hire the right staff.

The authors have nothing to disclose.
[a] Withers Bergman LLP, Private Client and Tax Team, 157 Church Street, 12th Floor, New Haven, CT 06510-2100, USA; [b] Hofstra University Donald and Barbara Zucker School of Medicine; [c] Quinnipiac University Frank H. Netter MD School of Medicine; [d] Yale University School of Medicine; [e] HaloMedia Group; [f] TPIU Foundation
* Corresponding author. 669 Boston Post Road, Suite 8, Guilford, CT 06437.
E-mail address: kjleemd@aol.com

Otolaryngol Clin N Am 55 (2022) 161–170
https://doi.org/10.1016/j.otc.2021.07.013
0030-6665/22/© 2021 Elsevier Inc. All rights reserved.

The Organization

1. Implement an intuitive Web site.
2. Install a phone system that does not send the caller continuously from one extension to another.

Patients prefer to communicate with a compassionate, knowledgeable person.

People want to talk to a human unless artificial intelligence is advanced enough that the virtual assistant with a compassionate human voice can answer questions and think like a human. Such technology is not available yet, but the corresponding author has such an Artificial Intelligence system under development, Essential Decision Tree, and is recruiting interested clinicians to join.[1]

3. There are 5 categories of appointments: emergency (see the patient now), urgent (within 24 hours), semiurgent (within 48 hours), semielective (within 2 weeks), and elective (after 2 weeks). Leave one slot open for each category, except for elective. If you leave too many open slots and they are not filled, you may slow down building your practice. If there are no open slots, double book. You can adjust this. The bottom line is not to make the patient wait long for an appointment.
4. Give clear and simple directions to your building and to your office. Give clear directions for convenient parking and be sure the parking attendant is as compassionate and knowledgeable as your staff.
5. Have a compassionate, cheerful, knowledgeable receptionist to welcome and help the patient. Make sure the paperwork is intuitive.
6. Anyone representing you from your office or the hospital should be knowledgeable about your specialty and about that patient.
7. Whenever a test is scheduled, enter the date of the test and the date to expect the results. If you do not get the results, find out the reason and inform the patient and the ordering doctor.
8. A periodic staff meeting with the doctors and input from the staff is helpful. It gets everyone on the same page and builds morale. Keep minutes, not as a legal document but as a reminder of the instructions and to serve as a to-do list. At the next meeting or earlier, request a report on the status of the to-do list.
9. Take patient complaints seriously. Thank them and let them know you are appreciative and have taken steps to remedy the situation.
10. The office needs decorum addressing patients appropriately: keeping eye contact and showing genuine interest. Never embarrass the patients. Never say "I don't know" but say "I will find out and get back to you" and follow through. When staff have time off, there needs to be proper "handoff." When staff are leaving for vacation, there needs to be a specific person assigned to cover him/her. Before leaving, both should meet with the doctor.
11. All caregivers for a particular patient should communicate with each other, thus "one hand knows what the other is doing."
12. Outreach programs should be educational, not advertising. Give lectures to educate the public through clubs, schools, religious organizations, or media. Create a column with questions and answers regarding common ENT ailments.
13. Implement a sophisticated "back business office" to do the coding, billing, claims processing, and adjudicating reimbursements. Never write off anything in accounts receivable if the insurance company has underpaid the mutually agreed fee.

The larger the practice group, the more effective the relationship with insurance companies. Forming a Single Tax ID group is advantageous. That was the message in 2001 to 2002 delivered by the corresponding author during his presidential year of the Academy. Since then, there are now many such groups across the country, the ENT and Allergy Group in New York and a group in Southeast Florida. The corresponding author is working to eliminate "precertification" and "denial of claims."[1] Volunteers are welcome. There is software to makethe electronic health record more user-centric. Volunteers are welcome.

14. Appropriate utilization of ancillary services located within the practice is convenient for the patients and can prove financially rewarding for the practice. However, care needs to be taken not to do unnecessary tests/procedures. The safety of the patients and the staff is of paramount importance. A review of the current Stark laws by a health care attorney is a must.

15. There are generally 2 compensation formulae, one based on actual cash collected by the practice (cash model) and one based on "RVUs" (relative value unit), the effort put in by the physicians (RVU model). The RVU model is less precise and often leads to some unhappiness. The cash model is more straightforward. The RVU model recognizes the effort of the physician who renders care to the indigent, which is lacking in the cash model.

The cash model:

a. Equal in, equal out distribution to physicians. This appears to be a simple formula, but it is next to impossible to find different physicians working the same number of hours, producing the same workload, and having the same efficiency. Taking the total cash received by the practice, paying the overhead, and dividing the balance equally usually leads to unhappiness.

b. Unequal in, equal out can lead to more productive physicians leaving the practice.

c. Equal in, unequal out by paying the senior physicians for seniority leads to unhappiness.

d. Unequal in, unequal out seems to be the most sustainable model provided the overhead is paid in a fair way.

e. Definition of overhead: There is fixed overhead (eg, rent) and variable overhead (eg, supplies, human resources, and utilities). The busier physician incurs more variable expenses. One way is to pay the fixed overhead equally and the variable overhead proportionate to the cash received by the individual physicians. For simplicity, some groups just divide all the overhead proportionately; however, the busier physician pays more and may be unhappy. Conversely he/she can look at it that he/she is taking home more money. Physicians, like anyone, can be envious. The less productive physician may begrudge the busier physician. Because the overhead is paid for proportionately, the less busy physician can take comfort that more of the overhead is shouldered by someone else.

f. Besides overhead, there is the capital expenditure, such as purchasing a computed tomographic (CT) scanner. The accountant has a depreciation schedule, and so forth. The CT scanner produces revenue in the year it was purchased and for many years thereafter. Therefore, if it were to be paid for proportionately in the month it was purchased, the higher earner of that month may not be the higher earner 8 years later. It may be better to pay for the capital account equally. The accountant or the bank can investigate the pros and cons of leasing or procuring a loan.

g. Overhead insurance covers overhead expenses when a physician is disabled. If overhead is paid proportionate to the revenue received by each physician, there is no need for overhead insurance. The disabled physician has little or no revenue, thus his/her obligation to pay overhead expenses is negligible. The other physicians see the patients of that physician and collect the revenue. The physician should still purchase disability insurance to support himself and the family.

h. Certain expenses incurred by a physician that benefit only that physician, such as travel to attend a medical conference, airfare, hotel, registration fees, and so forth, are legitimate tax deductions. One physician may fly business class; the other may fly coach class. It is important to preserve the legitimate tax deductibility, but such expenses should be paid by only the individual physician incurring the expenses.

16. Other than in a solo practice or a practice consisting of spouse and children, it is usually not wise for the practice to own the office space. For example, say a doctor, with a few of his colleagues who started the practice early on, bought the office space. They charge rent to the practice. As the practice grows, the practice adds new physicians who cannot afford to buy into the building or are not offered to do so. The practice continues to charge rent to the practice. The money is accrued only to the owners of the real estate. Landlords like higher rent; tenants like lower rent. Thus, conflict can start. The retiring physician may want to sell the practice and ownership of the real estate, complicating matters.

The following will help the doctor to have a successful practice.

The Doctor

1. Remember what you told your pre-med advisor and medical school admissions committee, and how you felt at the "white coat" ceremony—you genuinely want to take care of the sick and injured, listen to them, answer them, explain to them in terms they can understand (use of diagrams and videos are helpful), allay their fears, comfort them, and be available, amicable, approachable, attentive to your patients. The above will help to build a successful practice.
2. Develop a system that allows you to concentrate on the patient in front of you.
3. Develop a system in which test results are brought to your attention ASAP and promptly relayed to the patient in understandable terms. No results can be filed without your approval.
4. Explain the pros and cons of the recommended procedure/treatment in layman's terms as well as alternative procedures/treatments with their pros and cons. A simple postprocedure guide is a must.
5. Have patients write down their symptoms and questions before the visit. Encourage patients to ask questions.
6. If there is any bad news, the doctor should personally deliver this.
7. If there are any untoward results, be honest, be clear, and apologize. A humble, sincere apology does not necessarily admit guilt or wrongdoing.
8. Delegate administrative duties to a well-trained staff. Be consistent with your instructions and protocols and develop a simple manual. Appreciate your staff. Give "cheers and jeers" in appropriate doses at the appropriate time. Never reprimand a staff member in front of patients or other staff, "get mad at the right person, at the right time, at the right dose." When you need to give a jeer, incorporate a cheer or two.
9. Develop an incentive plan encouraging your staff not to call in sick frivolously. If staff do not use their paid sick days, those days can be used as planned vacation or be converted to cash. For every quarter that staff do not call in sick, they are awarded an extra planned day off. An office is more efficient and creates less commotion if it is not faced with unexpected staff "calling in sick," creating less stress and achieving more "wellness" for the doctor and everyone else.

10. Develop a system to assure that you are kept in the loop on all your patients. One is less stressed out when one is in the know and in charge. Surprises bring more problems and stress. Dr Michael Crain, head of Quinnipiac University Zucker School of Medicine White Coat Ceremony, said that the industrialization (commercialization) in medicine leads to depersonalization, which can lead to burnout. Relating to patients heals that.

Steps (A) 1 to 16 and (B) 1 to 10 can help to decrease burnout as well as build a successful practice.

Be thorough, pay attention to details, check and double check, and make a checklist that you look at frequently. The bottom line is you want to be a dedicated doctor guided by the 12 A's, supported by a sophisticated back business office. Once you realize the above and accept connecting with patients in a warm manner, you gain satisfaction, gain self-confidence, become calmer, become less stressed, and gain wellness. With this karma, you can better handle family and personal life, achieving work-life balance. Your reputation gets out in the community, and your practice is booming. People greet you in the supermarkets, places of worship, restaurants…"Hi, this is my great ENT doctor." You have the satisfaction of being assimilated into your community!

In the following discussion, written by an expert tax and estate planning attorney, the corresponding author suggests that if there is harmony in the family, the Executor of the Will and the Trustees of the Trusts should be beneficiaries of the estate and not outsiders (independent trustees) who can prolong the process, incurring huge fees. You can also stipulate the maximum and/or minimum amount that the beneficiary can receive each year.

TAX AND ESTATE PLANNING

While building a successful medical practice, consider steps to protect your wealth and benefit family and charitable goals in a tax-efficient manner.[2] Acting now on tax and estate planning, rather than leaving affairs to be handled by family upon your death, will best capture your desires for your legacy and may provide savings in the near and long term. Structuring assets in certain ways may help avoid probate, obtain creditor protection for beneficiaries, and minimize federal and state tax costs of transferring wealth. "Transfer taxes" include the estate tax (tax on your estate), gift tax (tax on lifetime gifts), and a generation-skipping transfer ("GST") tax (tax on gifts and distributions to your grandchildren and beyond).

Our discussion is divided into 4 parts. Part (A) addresses an individual's core estate planning documents. Part (B) explains the benefits of certain types of trusts. Part (C) discusses retirement planning. Part (D) provides certain considerations and techniques for charitable planning.

Core Estate Planning

The planning documents you should prioritize are your Will, Revocable Trust, and Ancillary Documents. These items are revocable, so make sure to revisit these documents every 3 to 5 years, and especially after a big life event and/or the enactment of a new tax act to consider any needed changes.

Will

Upon your death, if assets were titled to you individually, these assets and your Will would be subject to probate. Probate is the process by which the probate court transfers legal ownership and retitles your assets to your beneficiaries. Assets that you retitle to your Revocable Trust (discussed later) during your lifetime can help avoid probate of these assets. Depending on your state of residence, the probate process can be very expensive. Importantly, if you were to pass away without a Will, you could leave behind property to unintended beneficiaries. Your estate could run up fees in probate court before your property even benefits your loved ones. A Will designates property to intended beneficiaries, names guardians for any minor children, and appoints the Executor (or Personal Representative), who would handle your affairs. However, because a Will becomes a public document in probate court, to handle probate efficiently and provide privacy to you and your beneficiaries, consider a pour-over Will. Upon your death, all remaining assets will be transferred and titled to a trust, such as your Revocable Trust.

Revocable trust
Unlike a Will, a Revocable Trust agreement is generally not a public document. You can identify your beneficiaries and desired bequests in this trust without public scrutiny. Keeping your beneficiaries' inheritance in trust may extend certain creditor protection to them that they would not otherwise obtain if they were given their inheritance outright. Besides privacy and creditor protection, a Revocable Trust can offer tax-efficient transfers of your wealth. Structuring bequests in this Trust can help eliminate or minimize estate tax. The federal estate tax rate is currently 40%. Depending on your state of residence, there could be a separate state level estate tax. Currently, each US person has a federal gift, estate, and GST tax exemption of $11.7 million, which is set to decrease in 2026 to $5 million (plus certain inflation adjustments). In creating your Revocable Trust, you will want to maximize the use of your remaining exemption by fully allocating it in the Revocable Trust.

Ancillary documents
Do not wait until something happens to you before putting in place your Ancillaries, for example, health care proxy, durable power of attorney, or living will. By appointing your spouse or other trusted individual as your representative or attorney-in-fact, you will have someone who can act on your behalf for your health/financial matters even in your incapacity. In the event you become the patient, you will want your wishes followed, as provided in your living will.

Trust Planning

After establishing your core estate plan, consider the benefits of additional trust planning. Although these are sophisticated, irrevocable structures, careful planning with your attorney and advisors may further wealth planning goals:

Irrevocable life insurance trust
Insurance can be an important component of any estate plan. Proceeds can be used as an income replacement or a legacy item and distributed income tax-free to beneficiaries. However, if you are the owner of the policy, such proceeds on the policy on your life would be a part of your estate. Consider establishing an irrevocable life insurance trust (ILIT) to own the policy and designate it as beneficiary. Structured correctly, you can fund the trust gift tax-free using annual exclusion gifts (you can currently gift $15,000 per person-gift tax-free), and the trust can make premium payments. Upon your death, the proceeds will be distributed to the ILIT, income and estate tax-free. The ILIT will dictate the distributions to benefit your beneficiaries.

Gift/sale to grantor trust
What if there was a way to "freeze" your estate, such that future appreciation would be removed from your estate (transferred estate tax-free)? Using a gift to a grantor trust,

you may be able to keep assets for your benefit, while providing family future growth and appreciation on those assets. Once a grantor trust is funded with a gift, there are opportunities to leverage the gift by selling additional assets to the trust in exchange for a promissory note. If trust assets yield a higher rate of return than the interest due under the promissory note, the appreciation becomes an asset of the trust, thereby increasing the amount of assets transferred without increasing the amount of the gift. A properly structured grantor trust can maximize the benefit of your available exemption, ensure that trust assets are not subject to transfer taxes while in the trust, and protect descendants against creditors for multiple generations. Consider planning with appreciating investments/business interests.

Grantor retained annuity trust
A grantor retained annuity trust (GRAT) is a "freeze" planning vehicle as well, especially useful if you have exhausted your estate and gift tax exemption. Although a gift to a grantor trust uses exemption, you can structure GRATs without using any (or minimal) exemption. You as the grantor transfer assets into an irrevocable trust and retain the right to receive an annuity payment for a fixed term of years. The retained annuity reduces the value of the transfer for gift tax purposes. When the annuity period ends, the assets in the trust (including appreciation) pass to your family and beneficiaries without transfer tax. However, unlike the grantor trust above, a GRAT is generally a one-generation planning vehicle for children. Trust assets may be subject to GST tax if grandchildren receive distributions. Consider planning with appreciating investments/business interests.

Qualified personal residence trust
A qualified personal residence trust (QPRT) is another "freeze" planning trust. You fund this trust with your residence. You transfer the future use and benefit of the residence now, at a discounted rate, and retain the right to use the residence rent-free for a fixed term of years. At the end of the rent-free term, the residence will continue to be held in trust for the benefit of your beneficiaries. If you survive the term, the value of the residence is no longer subject to estate tax. Like GRATs, this is generally a one-generation planning vehicle for children. Trust assets may be subject to GST tax if grandchildren receive property. After the QPRT term, you and your spouse may continue living in the residence, but would have to pay fair market value rent. Paying rent will further deplete your estate and transfer assets to your remainder beneficiaries in a gift tax-free manner.

Retirement Planning

Recognize opportunities available to save toward retirement. Make sure you revisit beneficiary designations to keep them updated.

You may be eligible to participate in a defined benefit plan or defined contribution plan. Possibly, if you own your practice, consider creating such a retirement plan for you and your employees. You may also be able to contribute to an Individual Retirement Arrangement ("IRA") or Roth IRA. In 2021, you can contribute up to $6000 (or $7000 if age 50 or older).

Currently, you can start making withdrawals from your defined contribution plans, IRAs, and Roth IRAs at age 59½ without penalty. Starting at age 72, defined contribution plans and IRAs will require a minimum distribution. If you do not withdraw the required minimum distributions, a 50% excise tax is imposed on the amount required to be distributed (but was not distributed).

Defined benefit
Also known as a pension plan, in the defined benefit, the employer provides for a specified monthly retirement benefit when you retire. The amount is predetermined based

on earning history and years of service. The employer will fund the plan and invest it for your retirement. Take note of any vesting schedules. Your pension income will be taxable when you receive your monthly benefit.

Defined contribution
Generally, the employee provides funding from deferring salary and can invest the funds. 401(k) (or 403(b) with nonprofit employers) are defined contribution plans. The defined contribution plan can be a profit-sharing plan, where the company contributes annually into the plan out of profits. Such a plan would contain a formula on allocating profits to each participant. Investments in the defined contribution plan are tax-deferred. You are taxed when taking distributions and includable in your income.

Individual retirement arrangement
You can fund an IRA with pretax or after-tax dollars. Funds grow tax-deferred before your withdrawal. If you do not exceed a certain income level or you do not have an employer-sponsored retirement plan, you may be able to deduct your contribution. You will be taxed when you take your distributions, which will be included in your income.

Roth individual retirement arrangement
You fund a Roth IRA with after-tax dollars. Funds grow tax-free and are income tax-free upon your withdrawal. There are income limitations to contributing to a Roth IRA. You can work around this limitation by "rolling-over" an IRA to a Roth IRA. Generally, this works by funding an IRA, paying taxes on contributions and gains, then converting to a Roth.

Charitable Planning

"Doing well" and "doing good" do not have to an either-or scenario. You can do well for yourself and do good for the community. The following are examples of tax-efficient strategies you can use to achieve your charitable goals, produce an effective wealth transfer to family, and/or reduce taxes through income tax deductions.

Charitable lead annuity trust
A grantor charitable lead annuity trust (CLAT) can optimize overall income and estate tax planning. Potential benefits of creating a grantor CLAT include an upfront charitable income tax deduction, a stream of payments to desired charities, removal of estate assets at little gift tax cost, and shifting wealth in a creditor-protected fashion to family. A CLAT pays an annuity to desired charities for a fixed term. This is the "lead" interest that generates the income tax deduction. Any remaining trust property after the term is the "remainder interest." The remainder interest will continue to be held in trust for the benefit of family and desired noncharitable beneficiaries. Effectiveness of the CLAT depends on earning investment returns in excess of the IRS rate used to calculate the present value of the annuity benefiting charity. Consider funding with cash.

Charitable remainder unitrust
A charitable remainder unitrust (CRUT) is the CLAT reversed. The "lead" interest benefits noncharitable beneficiaries, whereas the "remainder" interest benefits charity. On funding, you will receive an income tax deduction. The deduction will depend on the value contributed and lead interest of the CRUT, which is often structured for the benefit of you and your spouse (an income stream, typically, over your lives). Upon your deaths, the remainder is distributed to charity. A CRUT is considered

a tax-exempt entity. As a result, if and when trust assets are sold, no income tax is due. The entire sale proceeds are available for reinvestment. The CRUT, therefore, provides a deferral of income tax on the sale. Assets can compound on a tax-free basis. Consider funding with passive investments such as marketable securities.

Contribution of individual retirement arrangement distributions to charity
For charitable donations, consider giving IRA distributions to charity. If you are a retiree, age 70½ or older, you can donate up to $100,000 tax-free directly from your IRA. The qualified charitable distribution from your IRA would not be included in your income. If you were to otherwise take a distribution from your IRA and then make a donation, the distribution would be subject to income tax.

Donor-advised fund
You can establish a donor-advised fund (DAF), which is a segregated donor account at a public charity that is the DAF's sponsor. Contributions to a DAF will generate an income tax deduction and create a low-cost, grant-making vehicle. Although you as donor technically have no legal control over contributed assets, you can make grant recommendations to the sponsor, who may disburse funds toward your suggested recipient charities.

Private foundation
You can establish a Foundation, which is a distinct, tax-exempt entity. Contributions to the Foundation will generate an income tax deduction. A Foundation allows flexibility in charitable giving to recipients and structuring of the entity's governance. If your family is involved with the Foundation, the board structure can encourage younger generations to participate in the grant-making process. Building on your legacy, funds can remain within family control and investment for unlimited generations.

You have worked hard to create your practice. You deserve to have your financial success protected and your wishes honored. The above provides a survey of planning options, but is only a starting point of discussion. Note the above does not constitute legal or tax advice. Please consult an experienced tax and estate planning attorney to discuss and determine whether these options may apply.

REFERENCES

1. Available at: www.kjlee.world.
2. Available at: https://www.withersworldwide.com/en-gb/webinar-series-looking-ahead.

FURTHER READINGS

Lee KJ. Editorial. ENT J 2020;99(7).

Lee KJ, Lee ME. Otolaryngologist as a political leader? Otolaryngol Clin North Am 2020;53(4):685–99.

Lee KJ. Philosophy and reality of entrepreneurship. ENT & Audiology News. 2014; 23(1):40–2.

Lee LE, Yoneyhama C, Lee KJ. Real estate. In: Essential paths to life after residency. San Diego (CA): Plural Publishing, Inc.; 2013. Chapter 32.

Clary GJ, Lee KJ. How to work with software engineers in health information technology. In: : Essential paths to life after residency. San Diego (CA): Plural Publishing, Inc.; 2013. Chapter 31.

Lee KJ. How do you wind down. In: Essential paths to life after residency. San Diego (CA): Plural Publishing, Inc.; 2013. Chapter 22.

Lee KJ, Smith R. EHR/EMR: "meaningful use," stimulus money, and the serenity prayer. ENT J 2011;90(2):E25–8.

Das S, Eisenberg L, Lee KJ, et al. Meaningful use of electronic health records in otolaryngology: recommendations from the American Academy of Otolaryngology—Head and Neck Surgery Medical Informatics Committee. Otolaryngol Head Neck Surg 2011;144(2):135–41.

Lee KJ, Chan Y. Practical clinical guidelines go digital and "meaningful use.". In: Healthcare reform through practical clinical guidelines ear nose throat. San Diego (CA): Plural Publishing, Inc.; 2010. Chapter 35.

The impact of health care reform on providers (doctors). In: Healthcare Reform Through Practical Clinical Guidelines Ear Nose Throat. San Diego (CA): Plural Publishing, Inc.; 2010. Chapter 1.

A better way to implement EMRs. ENT Today 2010.

Usable EMRs and You. American Academy of Otolaryngology – Head and Neck Surgery Bulletin, March 2010. What to Look For in An EMR. Medical Economics, February 5, 2010.

Healthcare: affordable quality coverage for all. Otolaryngol Head Neck Surg 2009; 140(6):775–81.

Electronic medical records (EMR) – the train has left the station. ENTNews 2007; 16(3):45–6.

Managing Revenue & Expenses. Maintenance Manual for Lifelong Learning-Study Guide 11-24, 2002.

Lee KJ, Lee M. Universal healthcare: a bold proposal. Connecticut Medicine 2000; 64(8):485–91.

Mujtaba F, Sullivan E, Lee KJ. A method for detecting errors in discounted fee-for-service payments by insurance companies. ENT J 2000;79(3):148–52.

Lee KJ, Cobert-Alvarez J, Lee ME. Survival in the era of managed care. In: Advances in Otolaryngology—Head and Neck Surgery, Vol. XIII. Mosby, Inc.; 1999. Chapter 15.

How Global Capitation Can Calm Chaos in Healthcare Markets: American Journal of Integrated Healthcare April 1998. (This experience is now significant in the current Accountable Care Organization, "ACO" and how does ENT fit into an ACO).

Evaluating the lease vs. purchase decision. ENT J 1993;72:154–61.

Financial Considerations II
Loans, Debt Management, Saving, and Investing

Suparna Shah, MD[a], Brian McKinnon, MD, MBA, MPH[b],*,
Katherine Hicks, MD[b]

KEYWORDS

- Financial planning • Debt • Loans • Refinancing • Income • Savings • Insurance
- Investment

KEY POINTS

- The debt incurred from student loans is often a huge financial and emotional burden.
- Physicians should reduce costs as much as possible on the front end, remain educated throughout the process, and consider forgiveness programs or refinancing to optimize each person's individual repayment plan.
- Saving money, investing wisely, and obtaining insurance are integral to a physician's financial plan, which should be thoughtfully and comprehensively developed to ensure financial security for physicians and their families.

LOANS AND DEBT MANAGEMENT
Debt and Loans

There are 2 broad categories into which debts fall: secured and unsecured. A secured debt is one in which the borrower has acquired a loan that is backed by an asset that may be seized from the borrower if payments are insufficient. Two common examples are mortgages and automotive loans; if a borrower fails to make payments, the creditor may foreclose the home or repossess the car. Unsecured debt is not backed by an asset, such as credit card debt. In the event a borrower fails to make payments on these loans, he or she may be sued directly or a third-party debt collector may get involved. In general, the best strategy for debt repayment is to tackle the loans with the highest interest rates or most severe penalties first. The following is a brief summary of the most common loan types in the United States[1]:

The authors have no commercial or financial conflicts of interest nor any funding sources to disclose.

[a] Department of Otolaryngology–Head and Neck Surgery, Oregon Health Sciences University, Portland, OR 97239, USA; [b] Department of Otolaryngology–Head and Neck Surgery, UTMB Health, 301 University Boulevard, Galveston, TX 77555-0521, USA
* Corresponding author.
E-mail address: brmckinn@utmb.edu

Otolaryngol Clin N Am 55 (2022) 171–181
https://doi.org/10.1016/j.otc.2021.07.014
0030-6665/22/© 2021 Elsevier Inc. All rights reserved.

oto.theclinics.com

1. Credit card debt: This is extremely common and carries some of the highest interest rates of any loan type, often between 20% and 30%. In the United States, the average person owes $7027 in credit card debt.[2] This debt is best avoided altogether and should be paid off as soon as possible if it is incurred. In the event one is unable to pay off credit card debt in a timely manner, NerdWallet suggests meeting with a nonprofit credit counseling agency, consolidating credit card debts, transferring to a card with a 0% introductory interest rate, or consulting with a bankruptcy attorney.
2. Medical bill debt: This generally carries somewhat lower interest rates, but the principle charges accumulated can be overwhelming. It may be helpful to set up a payment plan or hire a medical bill advocate. One should avoid putting these charges on a standard credit card, given the high interest rates on these cards.
3. Business debt: This is often a necessity, particularly when one is starting a business. Small business loans or new lines of credit may be taken out to hire employees and purchase space and equipment. Apart from increasing the profitability of the company, one may also explore consolidation and refinancing options.
4. Automotive and home loans: These are secured debts that are structured similarly. Common approaches to tackling debt in these arenas is to trade in a car or downsize a home to a less expensive option.
5. Student loans: These are particularly overwhelming for those entering professional fields with lengthy, expensive educational tracks, such as medical and dental school. These students may also have substantial debt from their undergraduate education. The debt incurred during schooling is exacerbated by residency training, in which salaries are generally not sufficiently large to make substantial inroads in debt repayment.

Different Student Loan Types

There are 2 main categories of student loans: federal (or "direct") and private (**Table 1**). For the former, the US Department of Education is the lender, and interest rates vary depending on type of loan, type of borrower, and date of first disbursement. For reference, current interest rates for loans disbursed between July 1, 2020, and July 1, 2021, are as follows[3]:

- Direct subsidized or unsubsidized loans, undergraduate students: 2.75%
- Direct unsubsidized loans, graduate or professional students: 4.30%
- Direct PLUS loans, parents, and graduate or professional students: 5.30%

Table 1			
Types of student loans for undergraduate and graduate/professional students			
Type of Student	**Direct Subsidized**	**Direct Unsubsidized**	**Direct PLUS**
Undergraduate	May borrow between $5500 and $12,500 per year, depending on year in school and dependency status		Parent of dependent undergraduate may borrow to cover remainder of dependent's education costs not covered by other aid, as determined by school
Graduate or Professional	Not eligible	May borrow up to $20,500 per year	Student may borrow to cover remainder of education costs not covered by other aid, as determined by school

Federal loans offer the benefit of various income-based repayment plans, which are a prudent option while in training. Perhaps the most attractive feature of these loans is that they are eligible for loan forgiveness programs, which generally requires consolidation. During this process, the interest rates of each loan are averaged and rounded up to the nearest one-eighth of a point to compute the new interest rate. Given the advantages of income-based repayment plans and options for loan forgiveness, most medical students maximize the amount of federal loans that they borrow before applying for private loans.[4,5]

There are 4 primary types of federal loans:

1. Direct subsidized loans: available to undergraduate students who demonstrate a need for financial assistance in covering the cost of higher education. The amount that may be borrowed is determined by the institution and does not exceed a student's financial need. For these loans, interest is paid by the US Department of Education if a student is in school (>50% of the time), in a deferment period, or within 6 months of graduation.
2. Direct unsubsidized loans: available to undergraduate and graduate students and do not carry the requirement of demonstrating financial need. The amount that may be borrowed is again determined by the institution and is contingent on the cost of attendance, as well as other financial aid that a student receives. The key difference between these loans and subsidized loans is that the student is responsible for paying interest that accrues on unsubsidized loans at all times. All interest that is not paid during periods of deferment or forbearance accumulates and is capitalized, meaning the interest is added to the principal amount of the loan.
3. Direct PLUS loans: available to graduate or professional students and parents of dependent undergraduate students to pay for education-related expenses that are not covered by other financial aid. There is no need to demonstrate financial need; however, a satisfactory credit rating is necessary.
4. Direct consolidation loans: represent the consolidation of all eligible federal loans into one loan with a single loan servicer.

Should a student require additional loans beyond the maximum federal loan amount, they would then apply for private loans. Students attending some foreign medical schools may not qualify for federal student loans and would thus rely solely on private loans. In contrast to federal loans, private loans may be refinanced with private lenders, often at a significantly reduced interest rate.[5]

Minimizing and Managing Loans

Before considering loans, an applicant should seek out and apply for financial aid, grants, and scholarships. A list of these resources is available through the Association of American Medical Colleges (AAMC).[6] After these options have been used to the greatest extent possible, the next step is applying for loans to cover the remainder of costs.

Minimizing the amount of student loans is the first step toward optimizing loan management. On the front end, the application process can be quite expensive; researching admission criteria and being selective with the schools one applies to can save thousands of dollars.[7]

An essential step in navigating the student loan process is being educated and staying informed on the process and any relevant changes to it. In practice, this is very difficult because students are frequently overwhelmed and busy studying medical information and have little time to dedicate to learning about financial management. Few schools have made financial literacy a required component of their education. The vast majority do not have any time in their curriculum or advising that is dedicated to financial management. The AAMC offers a program called "FIRST" (Financial Information, Resources, Services, and Tools), which features informative videos and webinars on prudent loan management, as well as a tool called Med-Loans Organizer and Calculator, developed to help medical students and residents track loans and model various repayment strategies.[8] An essential component of loan management entails appropriate utilization of income-based repayment plans and loan forgiveness programs.

Loan Repayment

Generally, the expectation is to make full, on-time payments. If someone is experiencing difficulty making payments, it is best to reach out to the lender to explore options for reducing or postponing payments. When in a financial position to begin paying off loans, it is best to start with the loans carrying the highest interest rate. Credit card interest rates are notoriously high, and these should always be paid off first.

Two unique components of federal student loan repayment are income-based repayment plans and loan forgiveness programs, which are not available for private student loans. Income-driven repayment plans are calculated based on a borrower's discretionary income and family size.

Through the US Department of Education, there are 4 options for income-driven repayment, namely income-based repayment, income-contingent repayment, pay as you earn (PAYE), and revised PAYE plans. Although these are all income-driven, they differ from each other in several key areas[9]:

- Qualifying loan types (some loan types qualify only after being consolidated)[10]
- Advantages of plan
- Monthly payment calculation
- Repayment term
- Borrower eligibility requirements
- Public service loan forgiveness qualification

However, these loans do share several key features, including forgiveness of remaining balance at the end of the repayment period and the option for decreased or deferred payments during times of economic hardship. Each program requires annual recertification of income and family size so that monthly payments may be adjusted accordingly. Payments made under income-driven repayment plans may qualify for the Public Service Loan Forgiveness program. The AAMC's Web site section on loan repayment options features a downloadable chart summarizing the key features of all income-driven plans, as well as 3 traditional plans.[11] This chart represents a prudent starting point for someone considering which loans to consider and which repayment plan to pursue.

Loan Forgiveness Programs

There are several avenues that may be pursued to decrease or eliminate debt that is owed. Working for nonprofit or government facilities, for the military, or in underserved areas may reduce or eliminate medical school debt. Several of these programs are dedicated only toward students entering primary care specialties. In addition, there are many state-sponsored programs that residents should explore on matching.[7]

The program with which most young physicians are familiar is the Public Service Loan Forgiveness (PSLF) program.[12] Qualifying for PSLF requires the following:

- Physician must be employed full-time by a nonprofit or not-for-profit organization or by a federal, state, local, or tribal government entity
- Loans must be Direct Loans or other federal loans that have been consolidated into a Direct Loan
- Physician must be enrolled in an income-driven repayment plan
- Physician must complete 120 qualifying payments

Information on qualifying for and pursuing PSLF may be found at the Federal Student Aid Web site.[7]

Loan Refinancing

Residents whose specialties and/or employers render them ineligible for various loan forgiveness programs may consider refinancing through a private lender. There may be less flexibility with private lenders, but interest rates are often lower. Many private lenders have tried to mirror some attractive aspects of federal loans, including grace periods, options to use forbearance if necessary, and loan forgiveness in case of death or permanent disability.[13]

Historically, private lenders' interest rates for student loans were as low as 0.99% in the early 2000s, followed by a period during the global financial crisis in which refinancing was not offered. In 2013, refinancing services through private lenders were again offered. Current interest rates for private lenders range from 1.89% to approximately 9%, depending on the company and repayment terms.[14,15]

There are currently approximately a dozen major companies that offer refinancing services, and the competition has lowered rates and increased the availability of cash bonuses and other incentives. Credible (www.credible.com) is a company that serves as a marketplace for comparing multiple refinancing options side-by-side. The growth of the private lending sector has led to expansion of private lenders' services to better service those in need of financing. These services and benefits include consolidation services, cash bonuses, free refinancing, monthly payments as low as $75 for residents and fellows, discounts for autopay customers, unemployment protection, and, as mentioned, lower interest rates due to increased competition.[14,15]

SAVING AND INVESTING

Transitioning from residency to attending involves many changes, including a higher salary with significant discretionary income and new decisions to make about standard of living. How much should be spent, saved, or invested? During residency, financial management centered on covering expenses and saving money if possible; as an attending, investing becomes a real possibility. There are several considerations, as outlined in the following.

Expenses and Salary Allocation

How much of one's salary should be allocated toward monthly expenses, such as housing, transportation, food, and loans? The 50/30/20 rule is popular, wherein 50%, 30%, and 20% of income is allocated to living expenses, discretionary income, and savings, respectively. According to *US News & World Report*, the average gross salary for physicians in the United States is $206,500 (approximately $150,000 net), and those in surgical specialties frequently earn well above this figure. The average physician could easily modify the above rule to a 40/30/30 distribution. A physician earning $200,000 pre-tax would take home approximately $12,500 per month, allocating $5000 to expenses, $3750 to discretionary income, and $3750 to savings. Although expenses still represent the largest percentage overall, a larger proportion of a physician's income may be allocated to discretionary spending and, more importantly, savings.

Saving and Planning

How much of one's salary should be saved? One adage suggests saving an amount equivalent to income every 5 years starting at age 30. In this model, a person would have saved twice his or her income by age 35, triple by age 40, and so on. Assuming an average physician salary and a 35-year career (eg, employed from age 30–65), this rule of thumb would extrapolate to a total of $1,200,000, plus interest accumulated over that time period. Alternatively, a physician earning the average salary who applies the 40/30/30 rule would save $45,000 annually, resulting in a total of $1,575,000 plus interest saved over the same time period. These figures do not account for potential investment or interest that could be earned in a savings or a certificate of deposit (CD) account.

Often, an important component of a physician's financial plan is saving for their children's or future children's education. There are numerous savings plans designed to help in this pursuit; however, many are state-specific and may change over time. Thus, doing careful research is critical. **Table 2** summarizes several of these options.

Another very important component is retirement planning. One rule of thumb suggests that a person needs 80% of pre-retirement income to live comfortably. A physician earning a net salary of $150,000 should thus plan to save enough to provide $120,000 per year of retirement. Assuming that person lives 20 years after he or she retires, a total of $2,400,000 would be needed to maintain a similar standard of living, an amount nearly double to the savings calculated previously. Although social security may make up a small portion of the discrepancy, smart investing is essential.

Table 2
College savings plans

Options	Pro	Con
529 Plans	State-based tax-advantaged savings plan. Contributions are considered gifts from a tax perspective, and may be made by anyone. Beneficiary may be changed to other family members, and there is no time limit on use of funds.	Limited flexibility, as tax advantage is only for qualified expenses. 529 Plans are state based, which may limit benefit if attending out-of-state school. 529 Plan specifics vary between states.
Coverdell Education savings account	Funds may be spent on qualified expenses for elementary and high school, as well as college. Funds may be transferred to relative of the beneficiary.	Significant contribution and income limits. No state tax advantage. Funds must be spent by 30 y of age.
Roth IRA	Funds may be withdrawn penalty-free but not tax-free for higher education expenses.	Use of funds for higher education expenses may complicate retirement planning. Funds may adversely impact financial aid eligibility.
Brokerage accounts	Funds may be used for whatever you want, whenever you want.	Funds withdrawn will be treated as income, impacting financial aid eligibility.

Data from https://www.nytimes.com/guides/business/how-to-save-for-college, accessed May 15, 2021.

Investment and retirement plans

Although investing should be an integral component of a physician's financial plan, most physicians receive minimal if any guidance or education on this topic. Physicians recognize that saving money is important, and some may have casual familiarity with basic retirement plans, such as a 401(k). However, most are not well-versed in the different types of plans and the pros and cons of each. **Table 3** summarizes the key eligibility features of several common employer-sponsored plans.

Given the regulations for the various employer-sponsored retirement plans, a physician may not have much flexibility with respect to which plan he or she is eligible to participate in. Physicians in private practice may have more flexibility in this regard than employees of large hospital systems or academic medical centers. Their retirement plans may offer additional options, such as cash balance plans that allow more tax-sheltered retirement savings over and above the standard 401(k) plan. Regardless of which plan someone is enrolled in, the goals should be (1) to contribute the maximum amount possible annually ($19,500 for 2020–2021, with a catch-up provision for those older than 50), allowing for reasonable living expenses; and (2) to take advantage of any matching programs offered by the employer. After an automatic deduction has been calculated, it is prudent not to change it unless one wishes to increase the contribution amount.

Some companies offer pre-tax and after-tax options for these deductions. Pre-tax avoids taxation at time of contribution; instead, the distributions are taxed on withdrawal (required by age 72). In this case, the full amount of the original contribution *plus* growth of the investment is taxed. The after-tax (Roth) option taxes contributions at the time of investment; thus, any growth in the investment over time is not taxed on distribution of the account. There are pros and cons to both options, and individuals should consider their personal financial circumstances when deciding between them. The pre-tax option may be prudent for those currently in a high-income bracket who will have zero income

Table 3
Employer-sponsored retirement plan eligibility

Plan	Definition	Eligibility
401(k)	Qualified retirement plan that allows employees to contribute a portion of their wages to individual retirement accounts	Employees at for-profit companies
403(b)	Tax-sheltered annuity plan toward which employees may contribute	Employees at nonprofit or not-for-profit companies Government employees
457(b)	Deferred compensation plan that allows employees to defer income taxation on retirement savings into future years	State/local government employees
457(f)	Deferred compensation plan that may trigger different tax treatment than above	Top executives of nonprofit companies
TSP (Thrift savings plan)	Tax-deferred retirement savings and investment plan with savings and tax benefits comparable to 401(k) plans	Federal government employees

Data from: Types of Retirement Plans. https://www.irs.gov/retirement-plans/plan-sponsor/types-of-retirement-plans. Accessed May 13, 2021.

during retirement. However, the after-tax option avoids future taxation on the growth of the account, which may be substantial if wisely invested.

Other retirement options include traditional (pre-tax) and Roth (after-tax) individual retirement accounts (IRAs), which are taxed at time of withdrawal and investment, respectively. Other key differences are summarized in **Table 4**. These plans were originally introduced as an option for employees whose employers did not offer sponsored plans, such as a 401(k). However, currently, it is possible for an individual to contribute to both employer-sponsored plans and IRAs.

An investment strategy should take into consideration (1) how much risk an individual is willing to incur, (2) what types of investments will be made, and (3) how hands-on the investor plans to be. In general, one should diversify across many different types of investments early and modify this distribution over time. A diversified portfolio features stocks in companies that differ across the following parameters:

1. Industry type (eg, finance, technology)
2. Size (eg, small, large cap)
3. Location (eg, domestic, international)
4. Risk profile (eg, value vs growth stocks)

Usually, younger investors have a higher equity (eg, stocks) to fixed income (eg, bonds) ratio, with a gradual decrease over time. A frequently used formula is that percentage of investments in equity should be equal to 100 minus a person's age. Another commonly used investment strategy is dollar-cost averaging, in which the total amount invested in a particular asset is divided up into multiple periodic purchases. These purchases occur based on time intervals rather than on asset price. This strategy results in purchases being made at several different prices (and thus averaging out to a mean purchase price) rather than purchasing the entire amount at one price point. In many instances, it may be prudent to work with a financial advisor.

Finally, a physician in private practice should consider buying into his or her practice as an investment. A physician stands to make money when the practice or his or her shares of it are sold. Of course, this is most profitable in financially and structurally sound practices. Thus, investing in one's practice serves as further incentive to grow and optimize that practice on a daily basis.

Insurance

Insurance is a financial product intended to mitigate various adversities and hardships in life and their unforeseen consequences. **Table 5** represents a comprehensive list of personal and professional insurance options. Some forms of insurance (eg, business

Table 4
Characteristics of traditional and Roth individual retirement accounts (IRAs)

	Traditional IRA (Pre-tax)	Roth IRA (After-tax)
Income limit	No income limit	Income limits based on tax filing status
Maximum contribution	Total across all IRAs: <Age 50, $6000 and ≥Age 50, $7000	
Mandatory distribution age[a]	72	No mandatory distributions
Withdrawals taxable?	Yes	No

[a] Must take distribution at age 72 (age 70.5 for those who turned 70.5 in 2019 or earlier).

Data from: Roth Comparison Chart. https://www.irs.gov/retirement-plans/roth-comparison-chart. Accessed May 13, 2021, and Individual Retirement Arrangements (IRAs) https://www.irs.gov/retirement-plans/individual-retirement-arrangements-iras. Accessed May 13, 2021.

Table 5
Types of insurance

	Type	Description
Life insurance	Term life	Coverage is for a set period (eg, 10 y, 20 y, 30 y). At the end of the policy term, coverage is lost. Advantage: less expensive.
	Traditional life	Coverage is until the policy holder dies. More expensive. Variants: traditional whole life, universal life, variable universal life.
Disability insurance	Short term	Provides income protection for a 3-mo to 6-mo period, after a brief period (eg, 2–4 wk) of disability.
	Long term	Provides income protection for extended periods (years, or until retirement), after a prolonged period (eg, 3–6 mo) of disability.
	Office overhead disability	Intended to pay for business expenses during disability.
Business insurance	Business disruption insurance	Intended to pay for business expenses during period of prolong business closure (natural or other disaster).
Health insurance	Traditional	Examples include preferred provider organization, health maintenance organization, exclusive provider organization, and point of service.
	Dental	Coverage for dental care, which is usually not included in traditional health insurance.
	Short term	Temporary coverage during a lapse or loss health insurance coverage (eg, COBRA).
	Long-term care	Coverage for long-term care services (nursing home care, assisted living facility, or adult day care), not covered by health insurance.
Malpractice insurance	Claims-made	Coverage if the policy is in effect both when the incident took place and when a lawsuit is filed.
	Occurrence	Coverage for a claim for an event that took place during the period of coverage, even if the claim itself is filed after the policy lapses.
	Tail coverage	Extends claims-made coverage for lawsuits filed for an incident that occurred when coverage was in place, but after coverage has ended.

(continued on next page)

Table 5 *(continued)*		
	Type	Description
Personal and property	Home, auto, rental, etc	Coverage intended to protect from financial loss related to personal property.
	Umbrella	Personal liability coverage in excess of regular personal property policy coverage.

Data from: Member Insurance Programs. https://www.facs.org/member-services/join/insurance accessed 20210411.

and liability insurance) may be required by statute and regulation; others may simply be prudent (eg, health and disability insurance). The types of insurance policies one should obtain will vary with time, as will the magnitude of these policies. Maintaining an optimal insurance profile should be an important component of a person's financial plan.

SUMMARY

The student loan process can be overwhelming, particularly if one has other debts to manage concurrently. When planning for loan repayment, one should take advantage of the resources available to medical students, residents, and attending physicians. Equally important to paying off debts is starting to save and invest as early as possible. Although there are numerous strategies that may provide financial security in retirement, physicians should consistently save and invest, even if conservatively. However, an ample amount of time and research should go into financial planning, and physicians may not necessarily have the time or the motivation to do this. In these cases, it may be prudent to hire a financial advisor, particularly when making investment decisions. Consulting with other professionals, such as accountants and lawyers, may also be helpful in other financial planning activities, including managing student loans, setting up tax-sheltered accounts for future generations, and answering insurance questions. It is important to invest time in finding a professional who is reputable and trustworthy. Taking the time to find the right person will allow for peace of mind throughout the financial planning process.

REFERENCES

1. Pyles S. What is Debt and How to Handle It. Nerd Wallet. Available at: https://www.nerdwallet.com/article/finance/debt. Accessed June 24, 2021.
2. El Issa E. 2020 American household credit card debt study. Nerd Wallet; 2021. Available at: https://www.nerdwallet.com/blog/average-credit-card-debt-household/. Accessed June 24, 2021.
3. Federal interest rates and fees. Federal Student Aid; 2021. Available at: https://studentaid.gov/understand-aid/types/loans/interest-rates. Accessed May 1, 2021.
4. Loans. Federal Student Aid; 2021. Available at: https://studentaid.gov/understand-aid/types/loans. Accessed June 4, 2021.
5. Dahle J. Ultimate Guide to Student Loan Debt Management. White Coat Investor. Available at: https://www.whitecoatinvestor.com/ultimate-guide-to-student-loan-debt-management-for-doctors/. Accessed May 4, 2021.

6. Consumer and federal financial aid resources. Association of American Medical Colleges; 2021. Available at: https://students-residents.aamc.org/financial-aid-resources/consumer-and-federal-financial-aid-resources. Accessed May 1, 2021.
7. Budd K. 7 ways to reduce medical school debt. Association of American Medical Colleges. Available at: https://www.aamc.org/news-insights/7-ways-reduce-medical-school-debt. Accessed May 1, 2021.
8. MedLoans organizer and calculator (MLOC). Association of American Medical Colleges; 2021. Available at: https://students-residents.aamc.org/financial-aid-resources/medloans-organizer-and-calculator-mloc. Accessed May 3, 2021.
9. Income-driven repayment plans. Federal Student Aid; 2021. Available at: https://studentaid.gov/manage-loans/repayment/plans/income-driven. Accessed April 6, 2021.
10. Student loan consolidation. Federal Student Aid; 2021. Available at: https://studentaid.gov/manage-loans/consolidation. Accessed May 1, 2021.
11. Loan repayment options. Association of American Medical Colleges; 2021. Available at: https://students-residents.aamc.org/financial-aid-resources/loan-repayment-options. Accessed May 3, 2021.
12. Public Service Loan Forgiveness (PSLF). Federal Student Aid. Available at: https://studentaid.gov/manage-loans/forgiveness-cancellation/public-service. Accessed April 19, 2021.
13. Medical student loans: federal repayment vs. private refinancing. American Medical Association; 2021. Available at: https://www.ama-assn.org/residents-students/resident-student-finance/medical-student-loans-federal-repayment-vs-private. Accessed May 3, 2021.
14. Dahle J. Refinance medical school loans & consolidation guide. White Coat Investor. Available at: https://www.whitecoatinvestor.com/student-loan-refinancing/. Accessed May 1, 2021.
15. Dahle J. Refinance your medical school loans at a lower rate. White coat investor 2020. Available at: https://www.whitecoatinvestor.com/refinance-your-medical-school-loans-at-a-lower-rate/. Accessed May 3, 2021.

Otolaryngology Business Finance 101: Revenue Cycle Management, Insurance Contract Negotiation, and Benchmarking

Eileen Dauer, MD[a],*, Angela Lieser[b],
Amanda Ressemann, CENTC[b], Susan Koprek[b]

KEYWORDS

- Revenue cycle management • Insurance contract negotiation • Benchmarking
- Otolaryngology

KEY POINTS

- A basic understanding of how we get paid is fundamental to running a successful private practice or department.
- Revenue cycle management describes the steps a claim goes through from the time an appointment is made until the time the bill is paid and deposited in the business' bank account. Understanding the process and avoiding the pitfalls can pay dividends.
- Insurance contract negotiation is an increasingly challenging but necessary part of the business of otolaryngology; it serves as the foundation for reimbursement from private insurers.
- Benchmarking refers to the selection of metrics that are important to your business in terms of finances, operations, and human resources. Once these metrics are defined, they can be compared with prior months, years, or other similar businesses. The process allows for targeted improvements in underperforming areas.

INTRODUCTION

As otolaryngologists, we spend the better part of our early lives learning the building blocks to eventually become skilled clinicians. The foundation of science and math in high school and college gives way to learning anatomy, physiology, histology, statistics, and beyond in medical school. As we reach the pinnacle of our training in residency and fellowship, on-the-job training in clinic and the operating room are supplemented with reading and research that are generally specific to clinical scenarios and challenges. We then cram for our board examinations, and voilà! We are

The authors have nothing to disclose.
[a] St Cloud Ear Nose and Throat Clinic, P.A., 1528 Northway Drive, St Cloud, MN 56303, USA; [b] St Cloud Ear Nose and Throat, St Cloud, MN, USA
* Corresponding author.
E-mail address: edauer@stcloudent.com

Otolaryngol Clin N Am 55 (2022) 183–191
https://doi.org/10.1016/j.otc.2021.07.019
0030-6665/22/© 2021 Elsevier Inc. All rights reserved.
oto.theclinics.com

board-certified otolaryngologists. So where do we find the time and motivation to read about the business of medicine?

According to the latest American Academy of Otolaryngology Survey in 2017, nearly 58% of otolaryngologists are working in a private practice model,[1] which was higher than the 51% of private practitioners surveyed in the overall physician population in the same general timeframe (2018) by the American Medical Association (AMA).[2] If we are lucky, as we start our careers, we are surrounded by experienced staff members who are trustworthy and capable of helping us with this important work. Even in an employed or academic setting, as we advance in our careers, we will find ourselves called upon to sit in leadership roles for our hospitals, universities, and health systems that will require us to have a basic understanding of the business side of medicine. Therefore, we as physician leaders and business owners need a fundamental grasp of these processes to ensure the financial health of our business and/or department.

This article provides a foundational understanding of 3 key areas of the business of otolaryngology along with the pearls and pitfalls that should give the reader a primer in understanding these processes.

- Revenue cycle management
- Insurance contract negotiation
- Benchmarking the finance, operations, and human resource elements of the business

DISCUSSION
Revenue Cycle Management

How do we get paid? We may have a general awareness that we bill insurance for services rendered via Evaluation and Management (E&M), International Classification of Diseases (ICD), and Current Procedural Terminology (CPT) codes, but what are the steps involved from start to finish? These steps are called the revenue cycle, and ensuring it is done correctly is part of the revenue cycle management (RCM) process. Practice management software is available to help automate the process and is usually offered as imbedded or accessory software to complement a practice's electronic health record software. With the numerous financial challenges posed by the coronavirus pandemic, many practices found themselves in a position of razor thin margins and in need of maximizing their RCM efficiencies and reimbursement opportunities.[3]

RCM can be organized into several different steps, and the basic components are the following (**Fig. 1**).

1. Patient registration: When a patient is scheduled for an appointment, the phone scheduler gathers information from the patient or their referring provider, including demographics and insurance information, before the patient is seen at the clinic to verify insurance benefits. When the patient arrives at the appointment, the front desk staff then verifies the information that was previously entered to ensure its validity and to ensure there are no errors on the day of the appointment. Any discrepancies are discussed with the patient to correct them.

2. Insurance verification: This is a process that is carried out daily by accounts receivable staff to get an idea for the patient if the claim will be accepted or denied. This will give the patient a snapshot of copayments, deductibles, and out-of-pocket amounts accumulated at the time of checking the insurance so the front desk can collect on any balances that are due before being seen. This step helps to reduce the amount of delinquent patient accounts. Prior authorizations can also be done at this point to ensure proper reimbursement. Some vendors have this

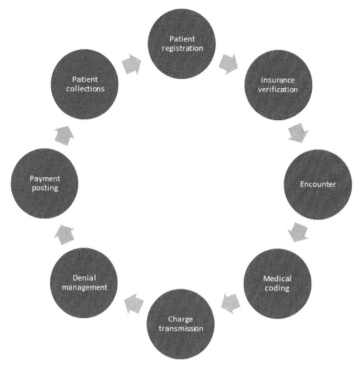

Fig. 1. Revenue cycle management steps.

feature built into the practice management software. If this feature is not included in your practice management software, you may be able to purchase a separate subscription with an outside vendor to complete this task before the patient's appointment.

3. Encounter: The preceding steps have led to this encounter, the step that we are most familiar with as clinicians, the patient visit. The encounter should give a clear record of the patient's visit, including prior treatments used for their complaint as well as the treatment plan moving forward. A diagnosis code is selected from the ICD-10 codes, along with billable procedures from CPT codes and a visit level code (E&M). These codes are added to the medical record, and charges are then pushed to the medical coding department to verify that the basic requirements are met for the selected services and conditions.

4. Medical coding: The encounter is reviewed, and appropriate charges are verified. This team should be experienced and have specific competencies in otolaryngology. Accuracy in this part of the RCM is critical. This claim can then be "pre-scrubbed" for errors such as missing modifiers, wrong number of units, wrong place of service, National Correct Coding Initiative (NCCI) edits, etc. Once this is completed, the medical coding staff pushes the claim to be transmitted to the clearinghouse. A clearinghouse is a go-between for the provider and the payer to securely transmit claims through an already established secure connection that meets the strict standards created by HIPAA. As most providers and payers use different software programs, the clearinghouse acts as a bridge for both the provider and payer to communicate through electronic data integration.

5. Charge transmission: Transmitting claims with accurate coding through your electronic data interchange (EDI) clearinghouse is the next step. There are 3 levels of errors that can occur at the clearinghouse level before the charge is submitted to the insurance company for payment.
   a. Scrubbing: The process of validating the combination of data presented in an insurance claim. The clearinghouse will run the charge through software that will validate the claim against Medicare/Medicaid/NCCI edits. Practice management software sometimes will let you add specific payer rules to your scrubbing software based on the insurance type to ensure a clean claim is processed by that insurance or you can purchase software that allows you to manually enter the claim information to verify if there will be any denials.
   b. EDI rejection: Invalid information held in the patient's record, such as incorrect date of birth, missing policy holder relationship, incorrect name spelling, and missing diagnosis code are a few examples of errors that will cause the claim to be rejected by the clearinghouse and sent back to the clinic.
   c. Payer rejections: Rejections by payers usually occur due to their payer-/plan-specific rules such as E&M codes, new versus established status, modifier use, and so on.
6. Denial management: Coming up with a process to deal efficiently with denials will be critical to effectively managing the revenue cycle. When denials are received, appeals are undertaken. As time and labor are finite resources, work on denials is prioritized according to payer, amount billed for the claim, as well as the date of the claim and the date of the initial denial. This process is done while keeping in mind the specific payer guidelines for timely filing. A fairly common timeframe for timely filing for private insurers is 3 months. After that period of time, an insurance company can deny payment due to delays. Large portions of potential revenue are at risk of being written off in that unfortunate situation. All insurers have a window where, if the claim is not authorized, it will never be paid.
   Identifying trends in denials will help inform earlier steps in the process of the RCM to boost the clean claim rate and reduce delayed payments and future denials from insurance. Although it can be a challenge (and sometimes will feel like trying to hit a moving target), putting in time in keeping up with medical policies from specific payers can be a worthwhile investment.
7. Payment posting: Accounts receivable staff should be able to provide an up-to-date snapshot on where each patient claim is in the RCM process; they monitor when payments have been posted to business bank account, and thereby ensure that delinquent patient accounts are followed up on and that denials are reviewed. This process will help ensure timely payment from both the patient and the insurance company. These staff also call insurance companies to track missing payments, nonpaid claims, and claim denials.
8. Patient collections: This can be the most difficult part of the cycle. The optimal time to collect from the patient is when they are in your office. Front desk staff should be well trained and comfortable with asking patients for these payments at the time of their clinic visit. Consistent messaging is used by phone schedulers at the time of appointment scheduling so that patients expect to pay these copayments at the time of service. For statement balances, statements should go out every 30 days to allow for optimal cash flow for the clinic.

Now that we have reviewed the specific steps of RCM, it is worth considering whether to use an outside service versus hiring staff to manage this process in-house. This is a very big decision for all clinics, and there are several factors to consider. First and foremost is clinic size. It has been suggested to have at least 0.61 AR staff members per FTE provider (or 1 biller/10,000 claims) to run an effective RCM cycle.[4] Having an outside company do this work can reduce your payroll and scheduling expenses. A practice must consider availability of staff with the appropriate expertise to do the required work. Even if you are inclined to keep control over this part of your business, when the labor market is tight, it can be exceptionally difficult to find the right staff to hire and give them appropriate training. If a large investment in time and training will be required to bring these staff up to speed on your business specifics, it may not be feasible.

Practices unable to hire the required number of skilled AR staff to effectively bill in-house may elect to outsource RCM to a third-party vendor. The biggest challenge with this decision is the loss of control of your accounts. These consulting businesses do have numerous staff with the training and skill to do the required work. However, these outside staff generally work on multiple accounts throughout the day and may restrict the amount of time spent on your account based on the negotiated contract. In addition, they may not be aware of the specific state rules for your insurance companies, which could result in denials or delays in payments. Aged accounts may increase, and you may receive more denials based on timely filing deadlines being reached. If a business does pursue a contract with a third party, it is typically advisable to negotiate a percentage of the claims they collect rather than a flat fee, so that they have skin in the game. Finally, consider hiring at least a skeleton crew of AR staff to monitor and audit the work that is done by the third party to ensure that the quality of their work lives up to the promises spelled out in the contract.

Insurance Contract Negotiation

While successfully navigating the RCM process helps to ensure you get paid, your insurance contracts will determine *how much* you get paid. Although there is no opportunity to negotiate with Centers for Medicare & Medicaid Services (CMS) for Medicare and Medicaid payment (their payment schedules are preset), private insurers are a different matter. It is important to negotiate and renegotiate contracts with these payers. Their primary goal is to make money for their shareholders. Their next responsibility is to the employer groups who purchase coverage and to the covered individuals in those plans. Their last concern is for the practices and providers who deliver care to their patients. The negotiation process with payers can be unpleasant at times, but if you do not take the initiative to aggressively pursue favorable contracts for your business, money will be left on the table.

The negotiation process starts with identifying the payers you will see the most. You may do this by looking at your historic trends and by identifying the carriers of the largest employers in your catchment area. Once you have identified your top payers, review your current contracts with those payers. Become familiar with their requirements for the practice, such as how many days they allow for a claim to be filed, to submit an appeal, to notify them of charge changes, and to complete the claim before it times out and is written off as a timely file.

It is helpful to designate one of your business office staff the task of negotiating contracts. This individual can partner with a physician. Whoever is in charge of contract negotiation should use a spreadsheet or similar organizational strategy to keep track of the payer contracts, the plan/strategy, the contract representative contact information, dates and terms of the contract period, and the date to notify of an intent to renegotiate.

To begin the process of negotiation (or renegotiation), the contract representative for the payer is notified of plans to negotiate new terms and communication lines are opened for exchange of information. Typically, at this point, a proposal is requested by the payer. To prepare an initial proposal, the prior year's codes are collated to highlight the top 20 codes used for the practice; this will include E&Ms, surgical procedures, audiological data, computed tomographic scans, SLP services, and other ancillary services to get a good cross section of the business. Next, the number of times each code was performed should be reviewed for the plan being negotiated. Relative value units (RVUs) are then compared from one year to the next, because they can vary significantly. CMS and RVS Update Committee (a multispecialty committee from the AMA designed to give physicians a voice in assigning RVUs) work together to create, review, and update RVUs. Congress requires CMS to review RVUs at least every 5 years, but there are slight changes annually.[5] If the total RVUs for one service increase, there will be an associated decrease in another area; for example, if the RVUs for E&M services increase, there may be a decrease in certain surgical services to balance.

Next, look at the conversion factor for the payer in the prior year. The conversion factor is the dollar amount that has been assigned to each RVU by the payer. The amount a payer will reimburse for a particular service is calculated by multiplying the RVUs with the conversion factor. The average payment for each service the prior year can then be calculated, and one can then determine what the request for the upcoming year should be. A letter is then drafted that highlights the achievements of the practice, the technology used to provide care, outreach locations for patient convenience, cost-saving measures that are used, and other positive attributes of the business to provide the payers with the best illustration of what is done for their members.

Once the request is submitted, the negotiations will go back and forth with the data updated each time until common ground is reached. Occasionally a plan will delay concluding negotiations or be generally unpleasant and unwilling to compromise. It is incumbent upon each individual practice to determine if it is best to walk away from a bad contract. When an agreement has been reached, the plan will forward paperwork for an authorized signature from the clinic and they will load the new fees in their system. On the renewal date, the new fees will become effective. Many plans will offer a 2-year contract rather than 1 year. These plans may agree to a higher conversion factor for year 1 if you agree to year 2, which will typically be lower or the same. Whether or not this is desired depends on the needs of the practice and the offer made.

Benchmarking

Benchmarking is the process of comparing metrics within one business between different points in time (internal benchmarks) or between one business and its peers (external benchmarks).[6] Benchmarking is a process, not an event; it is used as a tool for performance improvement. Benchmarking can take many different forms and can be tailored to the needs and goals of the business.[7] External benchmarks may require services from a health care benchmarking vendor to access relevant peer information. Some elements of benchmarking in hospital and health system settings will obviously be different than benchmarking for specialty clinics. For the purposes of this article, benchmarking examples are divided into financial, operational, and human resources (**Table 1**). Benchmarking is a complex subject, and we will just be scratching the surface of useful metrics that can be used in an otolaryngology clinic, without delving into the process of benchmarking. This list is not intended to be comprehensive, but rather to provide a primer on benchmarking. The reader is referred to numerous resources to further explore this subject, available through organizations such as the American Academy of Otolaryngology-Head and Neck Surgery

Table 1		
Benchmarking examples for outpatient clinic setting		
Financial Benchmarks	**Operational Benchmarks**	**HR Benchmarks**
Physician productivity	Appointment fill rates	Employee satisfaction
Income (gross charges, collections, net revenue)	No-show rates	Comparative pay analysis
Costs (total operating, staffing, expenses/cost of goods)	Number of days worked by physicians/APPs/audiologists/SLP	Employee turnover rates
Insurance claim Error Rate	Patient satisfaction	
Adjusted collection rate	Lobby wait times	
Payer mix	Access to appointments	
AR aging		

(AAO-HNS), Association of Otolaryngology Administrators (AOA), AMA, and Medical Group Management Association.

1. Financial benchmarks

There are several metrics that can be used to measure practice efficiency, both on the revenue and the expense sides of the ledger. Physicians, physician assistants, nurse practitioners, audiologists, and speech therapists are the revenue-generating part of the practice. Number of patients seen, revenue generated, and numbers of days worked can provide useful data in comparing productivity among these professionals, and this can be tracked in terms of RVUs or revenue/profit and can serve as a springboard for the calculation of bonuses.

Several payer-related metrics are also important to track. For example, AR awaiting insurance payments greater than 91 days should be at 15% or less. Generally, the goal is for insurance companies to pay for services within 60 days, as the practice should be concerned about having to write off the charges due to timely filing objections from the insurance company. Insurance claim errors that are not caught before the claim is sent to the insurance company should be less than 5% of total claims—every error delays payment and results in additional expenses to fix and resubmit. The adjusted collection rate, the amount we actually collect from insurance and patient payments divided by what we are allowed to collect from a contractual standpoint, should be above 90%. This tracking ensures accuracy in recording contractual adjustments and insurance denial reasons. Finally, payer mix, the percentage of revenue from private insurance, self-pay, Medicaid, Medicare, and so on enables a practice to ensure a healthy balance of payers and evaluate data for contractual amounts compared with what is received. This information can be particularly useful during the insurance contract negotiation process.

Expense-related benchmarks, such as staffing costs, are important to track. Personnel-related expenses should be kept under a certain percent of revenue (in our clinic, we try to keep that <70%). Targets can also be set for nonclinical FTEs (Full Time Equivalents). Benchmark surveys carried out regularly by the AAO-HNS Foundation and AOA can provide useful comparatives for setting goals for these expenses.[1]

2. Operational benchmarks

Operational benchmarks can be as varied as financial benchmarks, and which ones you track will depend on your patient population. One example would be tracking no-show rates of patients, which may inform policy on patients who are frequently late or do not cancel their appointment in a timely fashion. Appointment fill rates should be 90% to 95% to enable patient access while still maximizing clinic productivity.[8] Patient satisfaction levels can also be particularly important in this digital age in which unhappy patients have numerous online opportunities to share their less-than-stellar experiences with anyone who will listen. Similarly, patients are becoming less tolerant of waiting for long periods in lobbies and examination rooms, so it is critical for practices to find efficiencies to minimize those wait times. Finally, accessibility to appointments can have a big impact on keeping referring physicians (and their patients) happy with your practice, so number of days out for appointment availability is a useful metric.

3. Human resource benchmarks

Running an efficient business or department will also depend on your employees. Benchmarking coordinated between human resources and finance staff can help to predict the number of nurses, scribes, front desk staff, phone staff, and financial staff that is expected and optimal based on data from other clinics/industry leaders. Recruitment in a competitive labor market can present a challenge to finding the right number of employees, and investment in training is substantial. Therefore, it is critical to keep good staff engaged and satisfied. Employee satisfaction surveys, comparative pay analyses, and active employee retention programs all provide benchmark data to ensure that high-quality employees are retained and are performing at their peak. Employees will perform at their best when they feel they are doing important work, are valued, and are paid a fair wage.

SUMMARY

A fundamental understanding of the day-to-day operations of the business of otolaryngology is critical to the financial viability and success of our clinics and departments. Most of us have not had access to formal education or business experiences to draw from, and we must therefore seek out resources to educate ourselves on-the-job. In this article, we include insights into RCM, insurance contract negotiation, and benchmarking the business' financial, operational, and human resource elements to maximize the efficiency and financial well-being of the practice.

REFERENCES

1. Website: American Academy of Otolaryngology Survey. 2017. Available at: https://www.entnet.org/wp-content/uploads/2021/04/2017_SocioeconomicSurvey_v5.pdf. Accessed June 26, 2021.

2. American Medical Association. Physician Practice Benchmark Survey. 2018. Available at: https://www.ama-assn.org/about/research/physician-practice-benchmark-survey. Accessed June 26, 2021.

3. Website, Davis T. Tailoring your practice's RCM to changing times. In Physicians Practice. 2021. Available at: https://www.physicianspractice.com/view/tailoring-your-practice-s-rcm-to-changing-times. Accessed June 26, 2021.

4. Website. How Many Billers Do I Need? In Physicians Practice. January 1. 2008. Available at: https://www.physicianspractice.com/view/how-many-billers-do-i-need. Accessed June 1, 2021.

5. Website: Final Policy, Payment, and Quality Provisions Changes to the Medicare Physician Fee Schedule for Calendar Year 2021. Available at: https://www.cms.

gov/newsroom/fact-sheets/final-policy-payment-and-quality-provisions-changes-medicare-physician-fee-schedule-calendar-year-1. Accessed June 1, 2021.
6. Bisera C. First impressions and beyond: marketing your practice in touch points–Part II. J Med Pract Manage 2019;34(5):272–4.
7. Website: Statistically Speaking: Benchmark Report II, MGMA Insight Article, April 19, 2019. Available at: https://www.mgma.com/resources/financial-management/statistically-speaking-benchmark-report-ii. Accessed June 6, 2021.
8. Website: Watkins A, 7 Financial Reports your Practice Needs to Run. In Physicians Practice. 2019. Available at: https://www.physicianspractice.com/view/7-financial-reports-your-practice-needs-run. Accessed June 16, 2021.

The Value of Diversity, Equity, and Inclusion in Otolaryngology

Carrie L. Francis, MD[a], Cristina Cabrera-Muffly, MD[b],
Andrew G. Shuman, MD[c], David J. Brown, MD[c],*

KEYWORDS

- Diversity • Equity • Inclusion • Health care disparities
- Social determinants of health • Otolaryngology work force • Anti-racism

KEY POINTS

- Diversity, equity, and inclusion within otolaryngology benefits our patients by increasing patient satisfaction and compliance, improving outcomes, and better addressing health care disparities.
- Diversity, equity, and inclusion within otolaryngology benefits our practices by fostering innovation and higher performance when leveraging the unique talents of team members.
- Leaders of otolaryngology divisions and departments must invest in strategy to end bias in faculty hiring, development, research evaluation, publication practices, and retention.
- Recruitment and retention of a more diverse workforce withing OHNS will help decrease health care disparities and is a potential cost-saving measure for our society.
- A shift to greater cultural competency and cultural humility is necessary to achieve equity and justice while driving diversity of the physician workforce.
- To address these inequities, academic institutions must invest in study and strategy to end bias in faculty hiring, faculty development, research evaluation, and publication practices.
- Otolaryngology departments should prioritize D&I, making it integral to the mission and outputs (education, research, innovation, patient care).

DIVERSITY IMPACT ON PERFORMANCE

The racial and ethnic demographics of the United States are changing dynamically. Compared with 2016, by 2060, racial and ethnic diversity is projected to increase

[a] Department of Otolaryngology, Head & Neck Surgery, Workforce Innovation and Empowerment, Kansas University Medical Center, 3901 Rainbow Boulevard MS3010, Kansas City, KS 66160, USA; [b] Department of Otolaryngology Head and Neck Surgery, University of Colorado School of Medicine, 12631 East 17th Avenue Room 3110, Aurora, CO 80045, USA; [c] Department of Otolaryngology Head and Neck Surgery, Michigan Medicine, 1904 TC, 1500 East Med Center Drive, Ann Arbor, MI 48105, USA
* Corresponding author. 5101 Medical Sciences Building 1, 1150 West Medical Center Drive, SPC 5604, Ann Arbor, MI 48109-5604.
E-mail address: davidjb@med.umich.edu

Otolaryngol Clin N Am 55 (2022) 193–203
https://doi.org/10.1016/j.otc.2021.07.017
0030-6665/22/© 2021 Elsevier Inc. All rights reserved.

for Black or African American (13.3% to 15%), Asian (5.7% to 9.1%), Hispanic (17.8% to 27.5%), and multiracial individuals (2.6% to 6.2%). Multiracial individuals are projected to be the fastest growing racial or ethnic group. The non-Hispanic White population is projected to decrease from 61.3% to 44.3%, and thus, the United States will ultimately be a majority minority country.[1]

This rich diversity in our country reflects the future of our patients, learners, and workforce. Intentional and active incorporation of diversity, equity, and inclusion principles will allow everyone to thrive in health care, provide educational opportunities, and lead to job advancement. Our shared moral imperative to be leaders in promoting health regardless of race, creed, or color must reflect our common humanity. But it must also recognize existing inherent inequality and unfairness. As a recent Journal of the American Medical Association perspective opined, "when the fabric of communities upon which health depends is torn, then healers are called to mend it."

In addition to the moral and ethical obligation, diversity will actually make your team better. Diverse teams outperform homogeneous teams when addressing complex tasks because diversity fosters innovation, and diversity and inclusion (D&I) leads to higher quality performance by leveraging the unique talents of the team members to reach a higher level of excellence.[2]

Otolaryngology can learn diversity, equity, and inclusion lessons from the business world. When women represent more than 30% of the executives in a company, the overall performance was greater than that in those with 10% to 30% and even greater than that in companies with fewer than 10% women executives. Similarly, companies in the top quartile for ethnic and cultural diversity outperformed the bottom quartile by 36%.[3] Companies with more than average diversity have increased revenue secondary to innovations and services offered.[4]

Crisp and Turner state there are beneficial psychological and cognitive gains when we experience diversity beyond the stereotypical expectations and that this makes teams more tolerant and creative and improves both group and individual performance.[5] Diverse medical teams with cultural competence boost patient satisfaction and compliance, increase the accuracy of clinical decisions, and improve health outcomes.[6] Within otolaryngology, a diverse workforce would reach broader segments of the population. The expertise and experience of a diverse otolaryngology workforce would bring innovation and quality-improvement initiatives and foster stronger community health engagements for cancer screenings and hearing health services, to name a few.

In a study of Fortune 500 companies, including health care companies, Miller and Triana showed that boards with higher racial and gender diversity have higher reputations and more accurate risk assessments which leads to improved innovation from the collective wisdom and experience of a diverse group of individuals.[7] D&I of various perspectives disrupts the groupthink phenomenon and, thus, leads to a more ideal risk assessment.[8]

The presence or lack of visible diversity can impact one's feeling of belonging. Patients look for diversity of physicians and staff, and medical students often judge photos on the hospital walls which frequently tell the history of medicine being a White and male dominated profession. The lack of belonging can lead to trust issues, imposter syndrome, isolation, and decreased performance.[9] Microaggressions are discriminatory statements or actions often against marginalized racial and ethnic individuals and implies that they are lesser and erodes belonging. Microaggressions impact individuals and groups and contribute to $450 billion to $550 billion in losses per year in the United States (Gallup Poll).

ETHICS AND EQUITY

In addition to the social justice and representative labor arguments toward diversifying the otolaryngology head and neck surgery (OHNS) workforce, another important consideration is its impact on minority and underrepresented patient populations. This health equity argument is based on evidence that minority patients tend to prefer and have better interactions with physicians from their own background.[10] In an era in which public metrics of patient satisfaction are scrutinized for both quality improvement as well as marketing, data demonstrating lower Press Ganey scores for race- and gender-discordant patient-provider dyads are even more important.[11] However, the narrative that such discordances sufficiently and broadly explain satisfaction scores is also flawed because these findings were disputed in a Veterans' Affairs cohort. A diverse health care workforce engenders a higher level of inclusiveness for all its members, and thus, dyadic comparisons, while intriguing, cannot tell the entire tale of why diversity is so important to the broader patient experience. Part of this relates to the logistics of modern health care in which patient interactions with myriad clinicians and support staff all color their narrative.

A specific example may be instructive. The importance of appropriate pain management has been a national focus, including recognizing disparities in both access to and perception of pain control.[12] Data clearly corroborate that broad racial and ethnic disparities exist with regard to pain perception, assessment, and treatment.[13,14] Minoritized patients disproportionately underreport their pain.[15] The fact that certain populations may be stigmatized as drug-seeking, while also underreporting their own pain, only adds to their vulnerability and risk of not receiving adequate pain control. Racial congruence among patients and providers influences comfort with pain management as well.[16] Opiate stewardship has rightfully become a paramount issue within otolaryngology; recent practice guidelines stipulate how to responsibly stem the tide of the opiate epidemic while still providing adequate pain control.[17] But we also know that with regard to adult and pediatric tonsillectomy, there are formidable racial disparities in postoperative pain management.[18,19] Recognizance within our field regarding the need to address these entrenched disparities is thus critically important.

Esthetic preferences in facial plastic surgery represent another perspective on this issue. As providers and patients may not always look alike, cultural awareness of concepts of beauty and appearance requires a diverse lens.[20] The facial plastics literature is rife with myths regarding how people with skin of color want to or should be treated, reflecting a fundamental lack of cultural competency as well as frank ignorance.[21] Cultural congruence in esthetic preferences requires attention to these details. Patients of African descent generally do not want a "Caucasian" nose, and surgical management of the lower third, as an example, is much more nuanced.[22] As another example, empirical data demonstrate that when considering the aging face, Black women may focus more on pigmentation and soft-tissue volume rather than on rhytids and laxity.[23] This represents a business argument for increased awareness and outreach as Black women represent one of the largest growing consumer groups for fillers and other facial injectables.[24]

Given the clear importance of diversifying our workforce, it is all the more concerning that OHNS has markedly low proportions of physicians underrepresented in medicine (URiM) compared to other medical specialties and that growth rates of URiM OHNS physicians do not mirror growth rates of the racial and ethnic distribution of the US population. Preclinical student role models and mentors with similar backgrounds are also important to recruit trainees with whom they may more easily relate.[25] In addition, URiM physicians in training are more likely to incorporate care for minority and underserved communities into their future practice than their non-URM counterparts.[26]

As leaky pipelines continue, underrepresentation of URiM physicians also affects who will become health system leaders.[27] A leadership team with a dearth of diverse voices is unlikely to make strategic and cohesive decisions that address the concerns of the broader population. The longstanding absence of diverse senior administrators risks propagating and potentiating the ongoing impact of structuralized racism and is deleterious for the workforce and those being served alike.[28]

Barriers to achieving health equity are largely tied to social determinants of health. In a landmark article, Bergmark and Sedaghat[27] evaluated social determinants of health within OHNS. Social determinants of health include social and demographic factors such as socioeconomic status, health insurance status, and race/ethnicity that influence development of illness, the ability to access medical care, and adherence to treatment. Patients with decreased access to care are less likely to have a primary care provider, which can then compound the problem when subspecialty care is needed. There are fewer medical care providers within minority zip codes, and a large proportion of racial and ethnic minority patients use a small number of hospitals in the United States, referred to as "minority-serving hospitals."[27,29] These hospitals, which are generally poorly resourced, are also less likely to have enough subspecialty trained surgeons to the population need. Disparities in health equity have only been magnified during the coronavirus disease 2019 (COVID-19) pandemic, when multiple factors, including higher rates of medical comorbidities, delays in access to care, financial constraints, and distrust in the medical establishment, have led to increased morbidity and mortality among URM patients.[29]

Health care disparities have direct and indirect costs, leading to decreased efficiency in the health care system.[30] A study by the Joint Center for Political and Economic Studies estimated that between 2003 and 2006 alone, eliminating health disparities for minorities would have reduced direct medical expenditures by $229 billion.[31] This does not account for the additional indirect costs of loss of productivity and losses from premature death. When patients present with advanced disease, there is not only the increased cost in terms of morbidity but also the treatments are generally more expensive.

As subspecialists, otolaryngologists may perceive that health care disparities do not directly or significantly affect our patient practices. While we may be somewhat insulated from the disparities seen by primary care physicians, we nevertheless have a direct role in mitigating the effects of social determinants of health. We propose the following examples, listed in **Table 1**, to demonstrate how disparities related to social situations present within otolaryngology. Each example is followed by potential costs to our patients and our society. By becoming more aware of how commonly social determinants of health affect care within our patient populations, we can begin to address these costs.

Recruitment and retention of a more diverse workforce within OHNS, while clearly a moral imperative, will also help to decrease health care disparities and is a potential cost-saving measure for our society. Even at the individual level, OHNS can use cultural competence with humility to build rapport with patients, review their office policies to improve the experience for patients of different backgrounds, and advocate for policies that improve health care access.

TOWARD A VISION OF JUSTICE

The year 2020 saw a collective social awakening to ongoing racial injustice and structural racism with the rise of a global pandemic disproportionately killing Black

Table 1
Examples to demonstrate how disparities related to social situations present within otolaryngology

Social Determinant	Example	Potential Costs
Socioeconomic status	A 75-year-old person with severe hearing loss cannot afford hearing aids	Social isolation
Health care access/insurance	A 60-year-old patient with squamous cell carcinoma of the base of tongue and no health insurance	Increased morbidity; mortality
Language and literacy	An 18-month-old child with recurrent acute otitis media whose parents are non-English-speaking with poor health literacy	Language delay; increased morbidity
Transportation	A 30-year-old person with no way to get to the hospital for scheduled surgical repair of a mandible fracture	Prolonged disability
Secure housing	A 45-year-old person with acute sinusitis who lost antibiotics after being evicted	Complications from untreated disease; need for higher level care
Race and ethnicity	Black male who is not offered all treatment options because of systemic bias	Increased morbidity
Public safety	A 50-year-old person with orbital floor fracture after assault in her high crime neighborhood	Vision loss
Social support	A 25-year-old undocumented worker with recurrent peritonsillar abscesses; family lives in another country	Loss of income; job loss

Americans, Hispanic or Latin Americans, and American Indian or Alaska Natives. While society reckons with the unequal impact of COVID-19 and racial injustice, many institutions released statements with various commitments to antiracism, closing the disparity gap and increasing the diversity of the physician workforce. We are at a crossroad where the opportunity to acknowledge and dismantle the ongoing legacy of racism in medicine looms before us. From a strategic standpoint, equity and justice in medicine moves beyond interpersonal discrimination and addresses the structural barriers that impact health care education and delivery. Equitable and just practices drive diversity, inclusion, and belonging.

D&I have measurable benefits. Business scholars have been studying organizational diversity for a decade or more and have shown that investing in diverse talent increases profits.[32] Newer studies are emerging in science, technology, engineering, and mathematics showing that organizational diversity also results in greater research innovation.[33] In fields that require complex thoughts and problem-solving abilities, such as medicine, diversity leads to nuanced reasoning, troubleshooting, and innovation.[32] Simply interacting with individuals who differ from the institutional "norm" forces the entire group to prepare more comprehensively, anticipate alternative viewpoints, and expect that reaching consensus will take time and effort. Social science scholars investigating the impact of group composition on problem-solving consistently demonstrate the benefits of diversity: Adding social diversity makes people believe that differences in perspective might exist.[32]

These outcomes are meaningful in the context of ongoing homogeneity in otolaryngology as White, able-bodied, cis-gendered, and male sex. Refining our thought processes and considering diversity in knowledge, experiences, and perspectives are critical to appropriately addressing the disparity in the distribution of disease, illness, and well-being. Disparities are downstream effects of structural determinants of health and socioeconomic policy decisions that uphold institutional racism, class oppression, and gender discrimination.[34] Studies show that racial and ethnic diversity in learners during training makes physicians more comfortable treating diverse patients.[4] Others suggest race concordance is a preference beyond geographic accessibility and increases higher levels of trust and satisfaction by patients.[35–37] There is no genetic basis to race.[38] Thus, there is a cultural shift that needs to happen in medical education and current practice. A diverse physician workforce and a shift in medicine to greater cultural competency and cultural humility is necessary to achieve equity and justice while driving diversity of the physician workforce. Both skills help care providers respect patients' values, bridge gaps in understanding patient concerns, and allow us to look beyond individual behaviors and understand the structural barriers that create the context for an individual's manifestation of health, illness, and well-being.[39]

As otolaryngology departments have launched antiracism and diversity initiatives, it is imperative that there is an analysis of our environment as well as a focus on health outcomes. Acknowledgment of historical and present-day injustice and systemic racism is a first step toward a cultural shift. Meritocracy is a deeply ingrained belief in medicine, and studies have shown that rigid beliefs in meritocracy can exacerbate inequality — the paradox of meritocracy.[32] When meritocracy is blindly prioritized, it is easy to believe that one is impartial. This can lead to a lack of monitoring or scrutinizing policies, standards, or norms that for decades have reinforced inequity and created an environment where there is unfair disadvantage among underrepresented groups and unfair advantage among traditionally majority groups. As a specialty, otolaryngology does not exist independently from the value-based social hierarchy that occurs in the United States. Social injustice can be perpetrated over time and across multiple contexts.[40] This includes active exclusion from the profession and professional development from residency and faculty recruitment to sponsorship and promotion and tenure. Groups traditionally URiM, especially Black/African Americans, remain less likely to be promoted even after controlling for percentage of time in clinical duties and years as a faculty member, measures of academic productivity.[32] Many have described these inequities as a minority tax, a considerable barrier that makes advancement in rank and leadership, among other successes difficult to achieve.[1] The "minority tax" describes the undue responsibilities and requests placed upon the few faculty who are URiM to participate in efforts designed to increase "visible" diversity and can impede career advancement.[40,41] Such examples may include mentoring underrepresented students, trainees, or faculty; participating in diversity efforts instead of traditionally career-promoting activities; and navigating the burden of symbolic racism and microaggression. Racially and ethnically underrepresented faculty are often excluded from medical research in funding, publication, and promotion.[42] A recent study reveals that underrepresented scholars were found to outperform their peers in novel research.[33] They found that underrepresented scholars' work is less likely to be promoted or result in successful scientific careers. Hofstra and colleagues found that underrepresented groups must innovate at higher levels to have similar levels of career success.[33] Scholarship from underrepresented faculty members is often undercited, and their contributions to novel research and innovation undervalued.[42] This plays a critical role in faculty hiring and evaluation, such as how research committees evaluate research portfolios, institutional pedigree, or advising/mentor lineage.

To address these inequities, academic institutions must invest in study and strategy to end bias in faculty hiring, faculty development, research evaluation, and publication practices. Recruitment and retention require intentional investment in inclusive hiring practices and faculty/personnel development. An analysis of Black and Hispanic/Latin faculty shows increasing underrepresentation in most specialties.[43] The experiences of minoritized faculty of color in predominantly White institutions and work environments have been well documented. Many faculty experience social isolation, active exclusion from the decision-making process, and imposterism.[44] Born from psychology, impostor syndrome is described by many to be a feeling of self-doubt or belief that one is inadequate or does not belong, despite evidence to the contrary. However, belonging is not automatic in a culture or environment that prioritizes conformity and standardization. Studies have shown that minoritized faculty of color need culturally responsive mentorship, peer support, and coaching to develop survival and success strategies.[44,45] Faculty search committees should require members to undergo unconscious bias training with continuing education on equitable hiring practices.[46,47] Building collaborative relationships with affinity organizations facilitate recruitment for underrepresented candidates.[46,47] Affinity organizations provide members access to shared resources and facilitate networking opportunities. Establishing clear job competencies and value of credentials before application review has also been identified as a best practice. In addition, Issac and colleagues reported that when women were at or above 25% of the applicant pool, bias was eliminated.[48] To address research and publication practices, Boyd and colleagues have proposed rigorous standards for how racial constructs are used and evaluated. They provide scholars with specific steps as authors, journal editors, and reviewers that address the ways in which medicine has (1) overlooked the role of racism in health and health care and (2) reified biologic race and individual attribution or behavior as the cause of disparity.[42]

Health disparity is also impacted by equity and justice in medicine and diversity of the physician workforce. Scholars have identified racism as a root cause of racial health inequity and social factors, such as racism, as a fundamental cause of disease through access and other mechanisms that impact disease outcome.[49,50] Jones and colleagues state that operationalizing health equity requires strategies that "value individuals and populations equally, recognizing and rectifying historical injustice, and provide resources according to need."[51] The authors go on to remind the reader that a critical understanding of both antiracism and antipoverty is required to achieve health equity.[51] The model combines an inclusive understanding of belonging and humanity with a gap analysis that centers marginalized interests. This link has been supported through publications that identify associations between bias and treatment recommendations, verbal and nonverbal communication, and maternal health.[52]

Why are systemic strategies needed to address D&I in academic medicine? Historically, strategies to address health disparity and health outcomes have narrowly focused on individual attributes and behavior. Yet, those interventions that require the most individual effort have the least potential to create widespread change.[53] Although anti-racism statements and diversity initiatives have become the norm in health care, we must ask ourselves if these commitments are making a difference in the experience of underrepresented learners, trainees, faculty, and the diverse patient populations we serve. Gill and colleagues[54] note, "there is a growing understanding of the relationship between the providers' work environments, patient outcomes, and organizational performance." So, it is imperative that our health care institutions and system leaders take ownership and build a mission that values equity, diversity, and inclusion as core elements of excellence; aligns with the institutional vision; and intentionally identifies and develops talent for leadership at all levels.[55]

Different strategies have been proposed to address disparity and achieve organizational change for underrepresented and marginalized groups. Gillespie and colleagues[56] published 10 best practices to achieve gender parity in global health organizations: (1) make D&I an essential element of global strategy, (2) tailor global D&I to fit local needs, (3) embed D&I throughout organizations, (4) multiply D&I impact via external partnerships, (5) maximize the role of employee resource groups (affinity groups), (6) maximize the role of diversity councils, (7) leverage D&I for innovation (and novel research), (8) leverage D&I for business development, (9) Chief Executive Officer (priority engagement), and (10) make sharing of D&I best practices a meta best practice (Adapted from Gillespie).

Eckstrand and colleagues[57] developed a framework with elements and processes for organizational change that affirms the lesbian, gay, bisexual, and transgender community in medicine. Their key elements for success are (1) organizational champions, (2) organizational priority, (3) depth of mission, (4) commitment to continuous learning, (5) commitment to D&I, and (6) organizational resources. Their key processes for success are (1) change management and information exchange, (2) action research, (3) relationship building, (4) values in action, and (5) leveraging resources.

Organizational equity, diversity, and inclusion strategies are difficult to address comprehensively. They are also inextricably linked to departmental D&I missions. On a smaller scale, otolaryngology departments should prioritize D&I, making it integral to the mission and outputs (education, research, innovation, patient care). Departmental leadership should affirm and include in the discussion and decision-making process all groups in an effort to maintain diversity, equity, and inclusion strategies. Sharing best practices and areas of opportunity through national governing organizations is necessary in developing a standard of ED&I. Finally, OHNS must invest in the pipeline and develop underrepresented students, trainees, and faculty. It is only through intentional, inclusive, and collaborative efforts that our ED&I missions will be achieved for the benefit of our patients, providers, staff, learners, and society.

DISCLOSURE

The authors have nothing to disclose.

REFERENCES

1. Vespa J, Medina L, David M, et al. Demographic turning points for the United States: population projections for 2020 to 2060. Population estimates and projections current population reports. Washington, DC: U.S. Census Bureau; 2020. p. 25–1144.

2. Page S. The diversity bonus: how great teams pay off in the knowledge economy. Princeton (NJ): Princeton University Press; 2019.

3. Diversity wins: how inclusion matters, May 19, 2020 report. Available at: https://www.mckinsey.com/featured-insights/diversity-and-inclusion/diversity-wins-how-inclusion-matters#.

4. Lorenzo R, Voigt N, Schetelig K, et al. The mix that matters. In: Innovation through diversity. The Boston Consulting Group; 2017. Available at: www.bcg.org.

5. Crisp RJ, Turner RN. Cognitive adaptation to the experience of social and cultural diversity. Psychol Bull 2011;137(2):242–66.

6. LaVeist TA, Pierre G. Integrating the 3Dsdsocial determinants, health disparities, and health-care workforce diversity. Publ Health Rep 2014;129(1_suppl2):9e14.

7. Miller T, Triana MC. Demographic diversity in the boardroom: mediators of the board diversity–firm performance relationship. J Manag Stud 2009;46:755–86.

8. Levine Sheen S, Apfelbaum Evan P, Bernard M, et al. Ethnic diversity deflates price bubbles. Proc Natl Acad Sci U S A 2014;111:18524–9.

9. Walton GM, Brady ST, Elliot AJ, et al. The many questions of belonging. In: Handbook of competence and motivation: theory and application. 2nd edition. New York, NY: Guilford Press; 2017. p. 272–93.

10. Saha S, Guiton G, Wimmers PF, et al. Student body racial and ethnic composition and diversity-related outcomes in US medical schools. JAMA 2008;300(10): 1135–45.

11. Takeshita J, Wang S, Loren AW, et al. Association of racial/ethnic and gender concordance between patients and physicians with patient experience ratings. JAMA Netw Open 2020;3:e2024583.

12. Institute of Medicine (US), Committee on Advancing Pain Research, Care, and Education. Relieving pain in America: a blueprint for transforming prevention, care, education, and research. Washington, DC: National Academies Press (US); 2011.

13. Green CR, Anderson KO, Baker TA, et al. The unequal burden of pain: confronting racial and ethnic disparities in pain. Pain Med 2003;4(3):277–94. Erratum in: Pain Med. 2005 Jan-Feb;6(1):99. Kaloukalani, Donna A [corrected to Kalauokalani, Donna A]. PMID: 12974827.

14. Anderson KO, Green CR, Payne R. Racial and ethnic disparities in pain: causes and consequences of unequal care. J Pain 2009;10(12):1187–204.

15. Abdelgadir J, Ong EW, Abdalla SM, et al. Demographic factors associated with patient-reported outcome measures in pain management. Pain Physician 2020; 23(1):17–24.

16. Grant AD, Miller MM, Hollingshead NA, et al. Intergroup anxiety in pain care: impact on treatment recommendations made by white providers for black patients. Pain 2020;161(6):1264–9.

17. Anne S, Mims JW, Tunkel DE, et al. Clinical practice guideline: opioid prescribing for analgesia after common otolaryngology operations executive summary. Otolaryngol Head Neck Surg 2021;164(4):687–703.

18. Bhattacharyya N, Shapiro NL. Associations between socioeconomic status and race with complications after tonsillectomy in children. Otolaryngol Head Neck Surg 2014;151(6):1055–60.

19. Bhattacharyya N. Healthcare disparities in revisits for complications after adult tonsillectomy. Am J Otolaryngol 2015;36(2):249–53.

20. Hicks KE, Thomas JR. The changing face of beauty: a global assessment of facial beauty. Otolaryngol Clin North Am 2020;53(2):185–94.

21. Alexis AF, Few J, Callender VD, et al. Myths and knowledge gaps in the aesthetic treatment of patients with skin of color. J Drugs Dermatol 2019;18(7):616–22.

22. Boahene KDO. Management of the nasal tip, nasal base, and soft tissue envelope in patients of african descent. Otolaryngol Clin North Am 2020;53(2):309–17.

23. Alexis A, Boyd C, Callender V, et al. Understanding the female african american facial aesthetic patient. J Drugs Dermatol 2019;18(9):858–66.

24. Burgess C, Awosika O. Ethnic and gender considerations in the use of facial injectables: african-american patients. Plast Reconstr Surg 2015;136(5 Suppl): 28S–31S.

25. Kendrick K, Withey S, Batson A, et al. Predictors of satisfying and impactful clinical shadowing experiences for underrepresented minority high school students interested in healthcare careers. J Natl Med Assoc 2020;112(4):381–6.

26. Tusty M, Flores B, Victor R, et al. The long "Race" to diversity in otolaryngology. Otolaryngol Head Neck Surg 2021;164(1):6–8.

27. Bergmark RW, Sedaghat AR. Disparities in health in the United States: an overview of the social determinants of health for otolaryngologists. Laryngoscope Investig Otolaryngol 2017;2(4):187–93.

28. Spector B. Discourse on leadership: a critical appraisal. Ch 5: (White) men named John and the persistence of bias. Cambridge: Cambridge University Press; 2016.

29. Burks CA, Ortega G, Bergmark RW. COVID-19, disparities, and opportunities for equity in otolaryngology-unequal America. JAMA Otolaryngol Head Neck Surg 2020. https://doi.org/10.1001/jamaoto.2020.2874.

30. Jabbour J, Robey T, Cunningham MJ. Healthcare disparities in pediatric otolaryngology: a systematic review. Laryngoscope 2018;128(7):1699–713.

31. LaVeist TA, Gaskin DJ, Richard P. The economic burden of health Inequalities in the United States. Washington, DC: Joint Center for Political and Economic Studies; 2009. Available at: https://hsrc.himmelfarb.gwu.edu/cgi/viewcontent. cgi?article=1224&context=sphhs_policy_facpubs. Accessed April 15, 2021.

32. Francis CL, Villwock JA. Diversity and inclusion-why does it matter. Otolaryngol Clin North Am 2020;53(5):927–34.

33. Hofstra B, Kulkarni VV, Munoz-Najar Galvez S, et al. The diversity-innovation paradox in science. Proc Natl Acad Sci U S A 2020;117(17):9284–91.

34. Hofrichter R. Tackling health inequity through public health practice. Oxford University Press, Inc; 2010.

35. Smedley BD, Stith AY, Colburn L, et al, Institute of Medicine (US). The right thing to do, the smart thing to do: enhancing diversity in the health professions: summary of the symposium on diversity in health professions in honor of herbert W.Nickens, MD. In: Increasing racial and ethnic diversity among physicians: an intervention to address health disparities? Washington (DC): National Academies Press (US); 2001. Available at: https://www.ncbi.nlm.nih.gov/books/NBK223632/.

36. Ma A, Sanchez A, Ma M. The impact of patient-provider race/ethnicity concordance on provider visits: updated evidence from the medical expenditure panel survey. J Racial Ethn Health Disparities 2019;6(5):1011–20.

37. Cooper-Patrick L, Gallo JJ, Gonzales JJ, et al. Race, gender, and partnership in the patient-physician relationship. JAMA 1999;282(6):583–9.

38. Yudell M, Roberts D, DeSalle R, et al. Science and society. Taking race out of human genetics. Science 2016;351(6273):564–5.

39. Metzl JM, Hansen H. Structural competency: theorizing a new medical engagement with stigma and inequality. Soc Sci Med 2014;103:126–33.

40. Ross PT, Lypson ML, Byington CL, et al. Learning from the past and working in the present to create an antiracist future for academic medicine. Acad Med 2020;95(12):1781–6.

41. Rodríguez JE, Campbell KM, Pololi LH. Addressing disparities in academic medicine: what of the minority tax? BMC Med Educ 2015;15(1):6.
42. Boyd RW, Lindo EG, Weeks LD, et al. On racism: a new standard for publishing on racial health inequities. Health Aff Blog 2020. https://doi.org/10.1377/hblog20200630.939347.
43. Lett LA, Orji WU, Sebro R. Declining racial and ethnic representation in clinical academic medicine: a longitudinal study of 16 US medical specialties. PLoS One 2018;13(11):e0207274.
44. Hassouneh D, Lutz KF, Beckett AK, et al. The experiences of underrepresented minority faculty in schools of medicine. Med Educ Online 2014;19:24768.
45. Williams SN, Thakore BK, McGee R. Coaching to augment mentoring to achieve faculty diversity: a randomized controlled trial. Acad Med 2016;91(8):1128–35.
46. Rees MR, Bracewell M, Medical Academic Staff Committee of the British Medical Association. Academic factors in medical recruitment: evidence to support improvements in medical recruitment and retention by improving the academic content in medical posts. Postgrad Med J 2019;95(1124):323–7.
47. Shubeck SP, Newman EA, Vitous CA, et al. Hiring practices of US academic surgery departments-challenges and opportunities for more inclusive hiring. J Surg Res 2020;254:23–30.
48. Dossett LA, Mulholland MW, Newman EA, et al. Michigan Promise Working Group for Faculty Life Research. Building High-Performing Teams in Academic Surgery: The Opportunities and Challenges of Inclusive Recruitment Strategies. Acad Med 2019;94(8):1142–5.
49. Link BG, Phelan J. Social conditions as fundamental causes of disease. J Health Soc Behav 1995;(Spec No):80–94.
50. Phelan JC, Bruce G. Is racism a fundamental cause of inequalities in health? Link Annu Rev Sociol 2015;41(1):311–30.
51. Jones CP, Holden KB, Belton A. Strategies for achieving health equity: concern about the whole plus concern about the hole. Ethn Dis 2019;29(Suppl 2):345–8.
52. Schnierle J, Christian-Brathwaite N, Louisias M. Implicit bias: what every pediatrician should know about the effect of bias on health and future directions. Curr Probl Pediatr Adolesc Health Care 2019;49(2):34–44.
53. Frieden TR. A framework for public health action: the health impact pyramid. Am J Public Health 2010;100(4):590–5.
54. Gill GK, McNally MJ, Berman V. Effective diversity, equity, and inclusion practices. Healthc Manag Forum 2018;31:196–9.
55. Smith DG. Building institutional capacity for diversity and inclusion in academic medicine. Acad Med 2012;87:1511–5.
56. Gillespie JJ, Dunsire D, Luce CB. Attaining gender parity: diversity 5.0 and 10 best practices for global health care organizations. Health Care Manag 2018;37:195–204.
57. Eckstrand KL, Lunn MR, Yehia BR. Applying organizational change to promote lesbian, gay, bisexual, and transgender inclusion and reduce health disparities. LGBT Health 2017;4:174–80.

Moving?

Make sure your subscription moves with you!

To notify us of your new address, find your **Clinics Account Number** (located on your mailing label above your name), and contact customer service at:

Email: journalscustomerservice-usa@elsevier.com

800-654-2452 (subscribers in the U.S. & Canada)
314-447-8871 (subscribers outside of the U.S. & Canada)

Fax number: 314-447-8029

Elsevier Health Sciences Division
Subscription Customer Service
3251 Riverport Lane
Maryland Heights, MO 63043

*To ensure uninterrupted delivery of your subscription, please notify us at least 4 weeks in advance of move.

Printed and bound by CPI Group (UK) Ltd, Croydon, CR0 4YY

03/10/2024

01040400-0020